W9-BSZ-412

Developing Agility and Quickness

National Strength and Conditioning Association

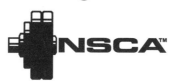

Jay Dawes
Mark Roozen

EDITORS

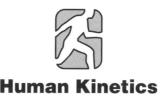

Human Kinetics

Library of Congress Cataloging-in-Publication Data

Developing agility and quickness / Jay Dawes, Mark Roozen, editors.

　　p. cm.

Includes bibliographical references and index.

ISBN-13: 978-0-7360-8326-3 (soft cover)

ISBN-10: 0-7360-8326-X (soft cover)

1. Sports sciences. 2. Sports--Physiological aspects. 3. Motor ability. 4. Motor learning. I. Dawes, Jay. II. Roozen, Mark, 1961- III. National Strength & Conditioning Association (U.S.)

GV558.D45 2011

613.71--dc23

　　　　　　　　　　　　　　　　2011025357

ISBN-10: 0-7360-8326-X (print)

ISBN-13: 978-0-7360-8326-3 (print)

The web addresses cited in this text were current as of June 2011, unless otherwise noted.

Developmental Editor: Heather Healy; **Assistant Editor:** Claire Marty; **Copyeditor:** Joy Wotherspoon; **Indexer:** Nan N. Badgett; **Permission Manager:** Martha Gullo; **Graphic Designer:** Joe Buck; **Graphic Artist:** Julie L. Denzer; **Cover Designer:** Keith Blomberg; **Photographer (cover):** Ben Liebenberg/NFL via Getty Images; **Photographer (interior):** Neil Bernstein, © Human Kinetics, unless otherwise noted; **Photo Asset Manager:** Laura Fitch; **Visual Production Assistant:** Joyce Brumfield; **Photo Production Manager:** Jason Allen; **Art Manager:** Kelly Hendren; **Associate Art Manager:** Alan L. Wilborn; **Art Style Development:** Joanne Brummett; **Illustrations:** © Human Kinetics, unless otherwise noted; **Printer:** Sheridan Books

We thank the National Strength and Conditioning Association in Colorado Springs, Colorado, for assistance in providing the location for the photo shoot for this book.

Human Kinetics books are available at special discounts for bulk purchase. Special editions or book excerpts can also be created to specification. For details, contact the Special Sales Manager at Human Kinetics.

Printed in the United States of America　　　10　9　8　7　6　5　4　3　2　1

The paper in this book is certified under a sustainable forestry program.

Human Kinetics

Website: www.HumanKinetics.com

United States: Human Kinetics
P.O. Box 5076
Champaign, IL 61825-5076
800-747-4457
e-mail: humank@hkusa.com

Canada: Human Kinetics
475 Devonshire Road Unit 100
Windsor, ON N8Y 2L5
800-465-7301 (in Canada only)
e-mail: info@hkcanada.com

Europe: Human Kinetics
107 Bradford Road
Stanningley
Leeds LS28 6AT, United Kingdom
+44 (0) 113 255 5665
e-mail: hk@hkeurope.com

Australia: Human Kinetics
57A Price Avenue
Lower Mitcham, South Australia 5062
08 8372 0999
e-mail: info@hkaustralia.com

New Zealand: Human Kinetics
P.O. Box 80
Torrens Park, South Australia 5062
0800 222 062
e-mail: info@hknewzealand.com

E4818

Developing Agility and Quickness

Contents

Introduction

For all athletes, the ability to quickly change direction is often the difference between success and failure. Virtually all sports involve whole-body movements that require athletes to rapidly and instantly accelerate, decelerate, or change direction in response to game situations. The reality is that in most sports, the ability to quickly change direction is more important than great straight-line sprinting speed. For this reason, many coaches and athletes are interested in finding effective ways to improve agility and quickness. The purpose of this book is to assist sports coaches, athletes, and strength and conditioning professionals in accomplishing this goal.

In 2002, Young, Jones, and Montgomery attempted to identify the most significant factors influencing agility performance. In particular, these authors divided agility performance variables into two main areas: change of direction speed and perceptual and decision-making factors.[7] Within these two main components, several subcomponents exist, as outlined in figure 1. Agility and quickness are complex sporting skills that include both physical and cognitive components.[1, 2, 3, 4, 5, 6, 7] An example is a kick or punt returner in American football waiting patiently to receive a ball who must immediately decide which way to maneuver through the defense to gain yardage. Or, imagine a point guard who dribbles down the lane and must determine whether to continue dribbling, pass the ball, or shoot. These are prime examples of how athletes must move and think fast to achieve lightning quickness on the field or court. Therefore, to maximize performance, athletic training programs must address both the physical and cognitive components of agility and quickness. Only then will athletes be able to truly bridge the gap between practice and competition.

Chapter 1 discusses factors that influence agility, such as change-of-direction speed, proper technique, body position, and physical attributes. It also covers the essential components of developing rapid force, high power output, and explosive movement, as well as how these fundamental attributes influence athletes' ability to achieve high-level performance.

Chapter 2 explores perceptual and decision-making skills (i.e., quickness factors), such as information processing, knowledge of situations, anticipation, and arousal and anxiety levels. Athletes with high-level agility performance are better at recognizing and capitalizing on task- and game-relevant cues that give them a competitive advantage over their opponents. In many cases, these skills separate elite performers from everyone else.

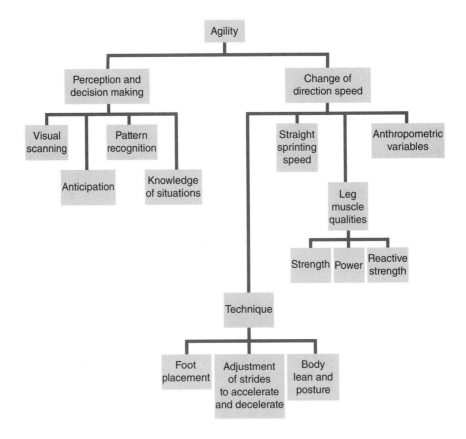

Figure 1 Components of agility.

Adapted, by permission, from W.B. Young, R. James, and I. Montgomery, 2002, "Is muscle power related to running speed with changes of direction?" *Journal of Sports Medicine and Physical Fitness* 42(3):282-288.

As with any training program, athletes must be physically prepared for the demands of training. Agility and quickness training is no different. Therefore, prior to the chapters with specific drills to enhance agility and quickness (chapters 4 and 5), chapter 3 discusses techniques to evaluate an athlete's readiness in detail. This chapter also presents methods for monitoring athletes' progress with both qualitative-movement assessments and tests that predict agility performance.

Chapters 4 and 5 present a wide variety of drills to improve agility and quickness. Many of these drills develop general motor programs and improve fundamental movement skills for future athletic success. These chapters also include suggestions and specific training drills that incorporate cognitive decision-making tasks into athletes' training programs once they have mastered the techniques. These unplanned, or *open,* drills require athletes to process information from the environment and to respond quickly with accuracy and precision.

The selected drills provide a solid base of information to assist in the development of athlete-specific and sport-specific training programs. Chapter 6 explores the basic foundations of designing agility and quickness programs. In chapter 7, professionals from a variety of sports share their personal philosophies on agility and quickness training and their favorite drills for improving sport performance at a variety of skill levels. The drills in this chapter add sport-specific training stimulus to the program, which better prepares athletes for the chaotic nature of sport and competition.

This book serves as a basic guide and resource for the safe and effective development of comprehensive training programs for agility and quickness. It is an absolute must-have resource for coaches and athletes who are serious about taking performance to the next level. It is loaded with invaluable training tips and information that the experts in this book have taken a lifetime to develop. The authors hope that athletes, coaches, and performance enthusiasts will gain an appreciation and a better understanding of what it takes to improve agility and quickness. Excellence is not an accident!

Key to Diagrams

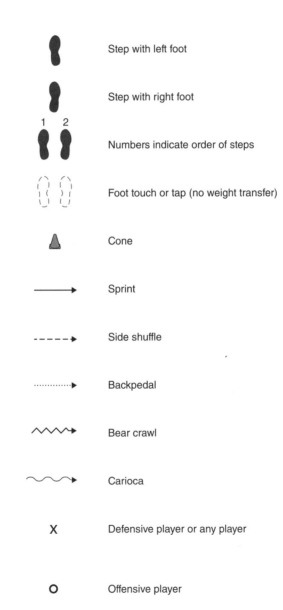

Step with left foot

Step with right foot

Numbers indicate order of steps

Foot touch or tap (no weight transfer)

Cone

Sprint

Side shuffle

Backpedal

Bear crawl

Carioca

X   Defensive player or any player

O   Offensive player

Factors Determining Agility

Mark Roozen
David N. Suprak

Most team sports, such as basketball, American football, and soccer, are characterized by rapid acceleration, deceleration, and changes of direction within a 10-yard (9 m) window.[45] Furthermore, court sports, like tennis and volleyball, also require multidirectional first-step quickness and changes of direction within a 4- to 10-meter (4–11 yard) span.[40] According to numerous coaches and sport scientists, an agility task is a rapid, whole-body change of direction or speed in response to a stimulus.[41, 53] Agility can be broken down into subcomponents made up of both physical qualities and cognitive abilities.[53] This chapter examines the physical qualities of speed, strength, power, and technique, as well as the qualities of leg muscles.

SPEED

Athletes who can move faster than their opponents have an advantage. For example, a faster athlete may be able to get to a ball more quickly than a competitor or may even outrun a pursuer. For this reason, athletes in most sports value speed highly. Speed is often measured by using linear (straight-line) sprinting over a distance between 40 and 100 yards (37–91 m). However, it is important to remember that in most sports, athletes rarely sprint more than 30 yards (27 m) in a straight line before they must make some type of directional change. Unless an athlete is a 100-meter sprinter, focusing a great deal of time and attention on straight-ahead speed may not result in optimum performance. On the other hand, since most sports require acceleration from a static state or when transitioning between movements, straight-line speed is still a valuable asset that athletes should focus on when testing and training for sports.

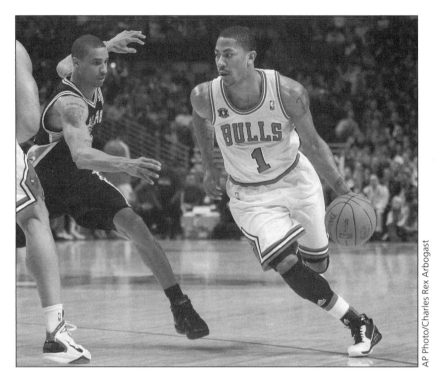

AP Photo/Charles Rex Arbogast

Derrick Rose accelerates past an opponent.

Linear sprinting is a physical skill that most people have performed since their second year of life with some level of proficiency.[22] For decades, many coaches believed that linear speed was mostly related to genetics and could not be significantly improved by training. However, appropriate training does improve running speed, even at the elite level. The combination of stride rate (the number of strides per unit of time) and stride length (the distance covered in a single stride) primarily determines linear speed. So, athletes can improve linear speed by increasing stride rate while maintaining stride length, increasing stride length while maintaining stride rate, or doing a combination of both.

Most sports, with the exception of track-and-field sprinting, involve short sprints (<30 yards) and rapid changes of direction, followed by rapid accelerations. For this reason, it makes little sense to focus a large proportion of training time on improving speed capabilities for athletes who will rarely reach maximum speed in competition. It makes more sense for these athletes to focus their attention on training to accelerate.[33] Acceleration is the rate of change in velocity, so this phase of sprinting is critical for changing directions as rapidly and efficiently as possible.

Optimal technique for linear sprinting in the acceleration phase involves four factors that maximize stride length and frequency:[34]

1. The body should have a pronounced forward lean that results in a lower center of mass. Consequently, momentum in a linear direction increases. This position initiates foot contact with the ground under or slightly behind the center of mass, reducing forces that cause an athlete to slow down or brake.[38]

2. When pushing off the ground during the propulsion phase, the foot touches the ground in a cocked position, with the ankle flexed upward at approximately 90 degrees (dorsiflexion) and the toes pointed back toward the shin. Once the foot makes contact with the ground, the athlete extends the hip, knee, and ankle simultaneously with as much force as possible (see figure 1.1). This movement is known as triple extension.[47]

3. During the recovery phase, the ankle of the free leg should be dorsiflexed while the knee and hip are bent, or flexed. This allows the foot to pass directly under the buttocks and a more rapid turnover at the hip.

4. The athlete should make certain to initiate arm swing at the shoulder with the elbow flexed to 90 degrees. He should work on swinging the arm forcefully backward to let the body's stored elastic energy and stretch reflex provide much of the arm's forward propulsion.[10]

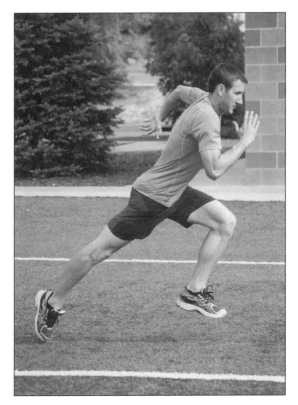

Figure 1.1 Proper technique for straight-ahead sprinting.

In the propulsion phase, the power output and rate of force development of the muscles that make up the hip extensors and the quadriceps muscles contribute to both stride length and frequency.[20] In the recovery phase of the sprint, the hip flexor muscles (located on the front side of the hip) and the hamstring muscles (located on the backside of the upper thigh) are the major contributors to stride frequency. The strength and power of the hip flexors are important factors in rotating the hip quickly from an extended position to a flexed position in preparation for subsequent foot contact.

The hamstrings have an important role as a multijoint muscle group. Because the hamstring muscles cross over both the hip and the knee, they are responsible for slowing down, or *decelerating*, the lower leg during the recovery phase in preparation for contact with the ground. At the same time, they also immediately transition to help the hip extend for the propulsion phase of sprinting.[55]

In contrast to straight-ahead sprinting, during backpedaling, the hamstring muscles are less active and the quadriceps muscles are more active.[15] Lateral movements involve more activity from the hip abductors than forward sprinting does. These muscles take the leg away from the body. Therefore, programs focused on improving agility performance should pay particular attention to developing strength in the hip flexors, the hamstrings, and the muscles that surround the hips.

Another important factor contributing to optimum speed is joint flexibility. If the hamstrings are excessively tight, athletes may not be able to bring the knee up as high during the recovery phase of sprinting, hindering hip flexion and speed. Furthermore, tight hip flexors may restrict the ability to extend the hip through the full necessary range of motion, thereby reducing power output during the triple-extension phase of propulsion. Proper flexibility of the involved joints contributes to movements that are more fluid and coordinated, resulting in longer and faster strides and greater speed.

STRENGTH

Strength is the maximum force that a muscle or muscle group can generate.[27] In most activities, athletes are unable to reach their optimal strength levels because of the speed at which they are moving. Strength is important, but so is the ability to use that strength to generate force. Force is calculated with the following equation:

$$\text{Force} = \text{Mass} \times \text{Acceleration}$$

Therefore, force can be altered by increasing the mass of the object being moved, increasing the acceleration of a given object's mass, or with a combination of both. Often coaches and athletes increase mass to improve force. However, as mass increases, or as weight is gained, athletes must be sure to maintain their ability to accelerate or move quickly. Gaining weight, even if it is lean mass, does not necessarily improve performance if it causes the athlete to lose a significant amount of speed.

Strength is an important contributor to agility and to athletic success. In agility development, increasing force to move the body more quickly relates directly to strength. Therefore, relative strength (strength in relation to body mass) is more important than absolute strength (the ability to move a given resistance regardless of body weight or mass). Important aspects of strength to consider when designing a program for improving agility include concentric, eccentric, and stabilization strength.

Concentric Strength

Concentric strength refers to the force exerted by a muscle as it shortens. Think of doing a biceps curl and bringing the weight upward. Lifting the weight requires a concentric movement of the biceps. Positive work (the force exerted against external resistance results in joint movement in the same direction as the force or in the opposite direction of the external resistance) also characterizes concentric muscle actions. An example is the push-off during a running, jumping, or cutting movement that is followed by powerful extension of the hip, knee, and ankle (this is *triple extension*; refer to figure 1.1 on page 3). Here, gravity works on the body to pull it down. However, with a powerful extension (straightening the ankles, knees, and hips), athletes can overcome the force of gravity and can more effectively run forward, jump, or make a cut. This will help them improve performance levels.

Theoretically, the more force the foot exerts against the ground during running or jumping, the greater the acceleration of the body mass will be. Likewise, the greater the force developed by the hip flexors during the recovery phase of running, the greater the forward acceleration from the hip. Increased force from the hip flexors also allows the athlete to position the foot more quickly for contact with the ground. This results in greater stride frequency during straight-line sprinting and directional changes.[13]

Scientific literature demonstrates a strong relationship between muscular strength and explosive movements, such as vertical[8] and horizontal jumping,[28] sprinting,[52] and agility[37] movements. The relationship between concentric strength and explosive movements is even more pronounced when relative strength is considered. Relative strength factors in the size and weight of an athlete. With absolute strength, if two athletes both squat 300 pounds (136 kg), they have the same maximum lift. If one of the athletes weighs

150 pounds (68 kg) and the other weighs 275 pounds (125 kg), the lighter athlete's relative strength is much greater than the teammate's. The heavier athlete would need to improve relative strength in order to be more explosive.

However, the relationship between concentric strength and explosive movements becomes less apparent when considering elite level athletes.[54] This suggests a threshold in strength at which further improvements in explosive movement performance are more closely related to the rate of force development (or in other words, the speed at which the necessary amount of force can be produced). Maximum concentric strength is especially important in the acceleration phase of sprinting.[52] Since acceleration is an integral factor in optimal agility technique, the role of concentric strength in maximizing agility performance is critical.

Eccentric Strength

Eccentric strength refers to the force exerted by a muscle as it lengthens. Negative work (the force exerted against external resistance results in joint movement in the opposite direction of the force or in the same direction as the external resistance) characterizes eccentric muscle actions. A simple example is lowering the weight back to the starting position during a biceps curl.

An athlete with high eccentric strength can quickly and effectively decelerate his body while maintaining dynamic balance in preparation for a directional change. The ability to decelerate the body quickly and with control is another important contributor to movements that involve rapid directional changes. Inadequate eccentric strength can slow deceleration and reduce the ability to quickly change direction. The relationship between eccentric strength and the ability to decelerate is exemplified by the movements in a stretch-shortening cycle (see page 11). In order to minimize contact time with the ground during a stretch-shortening cycle (and during agility-type movements), adequate eccentric strength is crucial for decelerating the body mass quickly so it can be accelerated in a new direction.

The ability to decelerate is important for both performance and for injury prevention. Athletes can attain the greatest amount of force during eccentric muscle action.[21] Most injuries occur during joint deceleration.[16] One of the main contributors to proper deceleration is eccentric strength of the involved musculature. If these structures are not strong enough to withstand force during movement, poor body mechanics can lead to improper body position, increasing the chance of injury. However, resistance and plyometric training of the eccentric strength allows athletes to augment their ability to decelerate body mass. This can translate into improved agility and athletic performance.

Stabilization Strength

Joint stability is an important and often overlooked factor that contributes to the effective application of force during agility movements. Agility training requires strengthening the muscles involved in stabilizing the trunk and the joints of the lower extremities. For example, when the foot touches the ground during a plant-and-cut movement, forces from the ground are transmitted up through the legs, hips, and trunk. If the musculature surrounding these joints and supporting the trunk are not stabilized by muscular contraction, then too much force may be absorbed or lost at these locations, slowing the transition from eccentric to concentric movements. This results in slow, inefficient movements and less than optimal skill performance.

An example of this is running a multidirectional cone-agility drill. If, due to inadequate core stability, an athlete lacks the ability to decelerate lateral forces when performing a cutting motion, he will take much longer to make a directional change. This potentially elevates the athlete's risk of injury. If a similar athlete who has the ability to stabilize the body and effectively change directions were to perform this same action, he may ultimately experience higher success and fewer injuries due to his movement proficiency, even if he were slightly slower.

Strength that optimizes stabilization is also important for muscle balance. For example, during hip extension in the push-off portion of sprinting, the gluteus maximus must contract to create the explosive movement that propels the body forward. However, the gluteus maximus also helps rotate the hip outward. Lack of control of this extraneous movement inhibits athletes' ability to propel themselves forward. To resist unwanted movement at the hip, the adductor magnus (a hip adductor that brings the leg back toward the body) must contract to improve the stability of the hip joint. This ensures that the force created by the gluteus maximus is used for forward propulsion of the body and is not wasted on other movements.[48]

In addition, the medial hamstrings (semimembranosus, located on the back portion of the upper thigh) and the lateral gastrocnemius muscles (located on the outside portion of the calves) aid in controlling undesirable movement at the knee joint during cutting maneuvers.[24] Both enhance the performance of these movements and reduce the risk for injury.[31]

Resistance-training exercises can enhance the strength and timing of the muscles' stabilizing contributions, including both bilateral (both sides) and unilateral (one side) drills, such as the following:[9, 23, 36]

▶ Multijoint movements, such as the back squat and forward, backward, and diagonal lunges

▶ Single-limb training, such as single-leg squats and other single-leg movements

▶ Explosive plyometric movements performed with correct technique, such as single-leg bounding and single-leg hops

Intermuscular coordination is another important aspect of muscular contraction that is closely related to stability during movement. Each muscle can send signals and information to other muscles in the system. The ease and speed at which they communicate relates to the activation timing of various muscles across a joint. Intermuscular coordination is important for running speed because if the hamstrings are not relaxed when the thigh is brought forward in the recovery phase of the stride, hip flexion will be reduced, resulting in a shorter stride length. This is especially clear in movements involving directional changes, where joint stability is of greater concern for the athlete. For example. soccer players who are more experienced display more coordinated patterns of muscle activation during cutting maneuvers

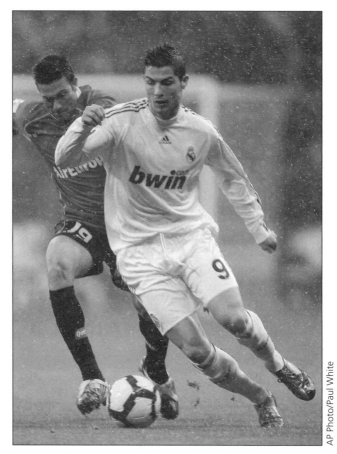

Experienced soccer players, such as Cristiano Ronaldo, display intermuscular coordination that allows for stability in speed and changes of direction.

than their less-experienced counterparts do.[42] Training involving acceleration, deceleration, and directional changes appears to contribute to improved intermuscular coordination and, in turn, better agility performance and a lower risk of injury.

Intramuscular coordination relates to an individual muscle's ability to improve motor-unit recruitment, rate coding (sometimes called *frequency coding*), and motor-unit synchronization.[39] The greater the number of motor units an athlete can recruit at a given time, the greater his ability to produce force. Likewise, with rate coding, as the intensity of stimulus increases, the rate of peak firing also increases. When these units are recruited quickly and in the appropriate sequence, an athlete can express this force over a reduced period of time, improving overall potential for speed.[39]

POWER

Power, defined as the rate of doing work,[14] is an extremely important concept in the expression of agility. It may be the most important determinant of athletic success.[43] Power can be calculated as follows:

$$Power = Work \div Time$$

In this equation, *time* means the period in which the work was performed. *Work* can be calculated with this equation:

$$Work = Force \times Distance$$

Power can also be calculated as follows:

$$Power = Force \times Velocity$$

In this equation, *velocity* is speed of movement in a specific direction.

The force-velocity relationship of muscle action shows that as the movement velocity increases, the force of muscle output decreases. This phenomenon is, of course, disadvantageous for athletes in sports that require both high force and high velocity. Examples of movements include starting, stopping, and changing direction. To train for this type of movement, athletes should focus on improving their ability to exert higher forces at high velocity. In turn, this will maximize power.

Keep in mind that athletes cannot effectively train for power by moving the body or the resistance slowly during training. As the previous equation suggests, power output can be improved by increasing force output, the velocity of movement, or both. Training methods for improving movement velocity differ significantly from those used for increasing force output, so a training program for agility development must incorporate both. One hypothesis suggests that to maximize muscular power, athletes must first maximize the magnitude of the force that a muscle is capable of producing (muscular strength). Then, they must maximize the rate at which this force is expressed (i.e., velocity). Building a base of strength is important for developing movement at higher speeds. This produces a higher output of power.

Rate of Force Development

Rate of force development is a characteristic of muscle-force output that is important for optimal functioning and closely relates to the discussion of power. This term is defined as the change in the level of force divided by the change in time.[25] To illustrate the importance of this concept, consider that it takes approximately 0.6 to 0.8 seconds to generate maximal isometric force.[56] However, athletes do not achieve maximum force during high-speed activities. In sprinting, for example, the foot contacts the ground for only about 0.1 to 0.2 seconds.[35] Therefore, the time constraints inherent in explosive activities, such as sprinting, jumping, throwing, acceleration, and changes of direction, dictate that force is developed quickly so that movement can occur rapidly.

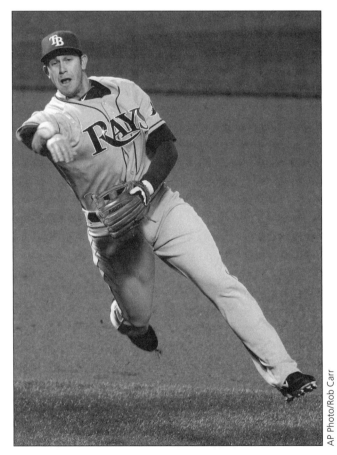

AP Photo/Rob Carr

Evan Longoria uses a high rate of force development to create a powerful throw quickly.

In these instances, the rate of force development becomes more important than the capability for maximum force.[51]

Part of the process of developing agility includes improving the rate of force development of involved musculature so that explosive movements can occur at higher forces. In turn, athletes can impart greater forces to the ground during foot contact. The rate of muscle activation is thought to be the primary factor influencing rate of force development.[30] However, other contributing factors may include patterns of motor-unit recruitment,[1] fiber-type composition, and muscle hypertrophy.[47] Performing explosive exercises, such as plyometrics and Olympic lifts (power cleans, snatches), at the right training load and intensity to produce proper speed of movement and force output can improve rate of force development.[18]

Stretch-Shortening Cycle

When required to jump in the air, most people quickly bend the hips, knees, and ankles, and then extend those joints. This is because rapidly stretching the involved musculotendinous structures (through an eccentric action) creates greater force and power output in a shorter amount of time during the subsequent shortening (concentric) action of the same structures.[29, 49] This process, known as the *stretch-shortening cycle*, is involved in most activities of daily living. Virtually all athletic skills that require maximum force and power output for successful performance use this cycle. Tasks comprised of sequential stretch-shortening cycles include winding up to pitch a ball, bending the arm before pulling a football from the arm of a running back to cause a fumble, bending down a few extra inches before getting up from a squat position, walking, or any other movement that involves rapid acceleration, deceleration, and changes of direction.

Three phases compose the stretch-shortening cycle: eccentric, amortization, and concentric (see figure 1.2 on page 12). In the eccentric (stretching) phase, the agonist muscles undergo a lengthening action as the athlete initiates the movement in the direction opposite to that of the intended movement. This phase is extremely important to the effectiveness of the stretch-shortening cycle, because this is where the muscle is stretched. Studies suggest that both a small magnitude (small range of motion) and high velocity of the stretching movement are important for maximizing its contribution to concentric force augmentation.[5, 32] By moving at smaller ranges of motion with great speed, athletes can achieve more recoil in the muscle and produce more force.

The amortization phase may be the most critical phase in the stretch-shortening cycle. It comprises the transition, or the time between the end of the eccentric phase and the beginning of the concentric phase of movement. The ability to switch quickly from the eccentric to the concentric phase of the stretch-shortening cycle is often termed *reactive strength*.[19] The concentric

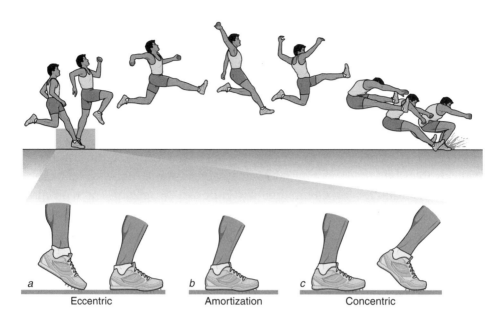

Figure 1.2 The stretch-shortening cycle in the long jump. The foot touching down to the end of the movement is the *(a)* eccentric phase. The transition from the eccentric phase to the concentric phase when no movement occurs is the *(b)* amortization phase. The start of the push off from the foot leaving the surface is the *(c)* concentric phase.

phase of the stretch-shortening cycle represents the time during which force application results in motion in the intended direction. In this phase, the previous eccentric action created increased force and power output of the agonist muscle-tendon units.

The stretch-shortening cycle has been studied for decades. The literature attributes the phenomenon to two main mechanisms: one of a neurophysiological nature and the other of a mechanical nature. The neurophysiological mechanism relates to the stretching reflex and the activity of the involved muscle spindles. When a muscle rapidly stretches (e.g., the rectus femoris and gastrocnemius at initial contact in a cutting maneuver), the corresponding muscle spindles, which lie parallel to the force-producing muscle fibers, also stretch. This results in a monosynaptic reflex, in which the sensory endings of the muscle spindles send a signal to the spinal cord about the change in muscle length. The spinal cord, in response, sends an excitatory signal to the corresponding muscle. These events result in the mechanical mechanism, which is a reflexive concentric action of the previously stretched muscle. This reflex may also be a protective mechanism against excessive stretching of the musculotendinous unit.

At this point, the length of the amortization phase becomes important. The stretching reflex occurs less than 50 milliseconds after a rapid stretch.[4, 5, 6] The amortization phase should be kept as short as possible in order to take advantage of the potential force increase that results from coupling the stretching reflex with active, concentric muscle action. In sport terms, visualize a boxer getting ready to throw a punch. If the boxer were to pull his arm back and hold it there for one or two seconds, the force developed would be greatly reduced. If the boxer were to rapidly *load the punch*, bringing the arm back quickly then explosively jabbing it forward (decreased amortization phase), the movement would be quicker and he would be able to generate more power.

Improved muscular efficiency also results from the storage of potential (elastic) energy in the musculotendinous unit. This involves the stretching of the series elastic component (tendon) and, to a lesser extent, parallel elastic components (intramuscular fascia) of the musculotendinous unit. Elastic

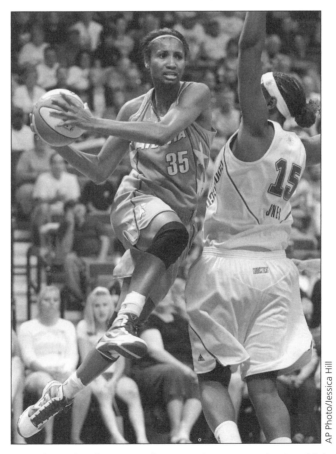

Recoiling muscle action increases force and power output, which allows athletes, such as Angel McCoughtry, to jump with force and power.

energy is stored within these components when the muscle is stretched. This energy is released shortly after it is stored, either in the form of the tissue recoiling to return to its original length or as heat. In sprinting, jumping, and cutting maneuvers, the stored energy is used in subsequent force production during the propulsion phase.

Once again, the length of the amortization phase has important implications here. The elastic energy stored in the series and parallel elastic components during the lengthening action only lasts a short time before it dissipates as heat. However, if the amortization phase is kept to a minimum, the recoiling action of the series and parallel elastic components couple with the active concentric muscle action, resulting in increased force and power output. If athletes rely exclusively on muscular contraction without prestretching, they will need much more energy to do the same tasks, and they would not be able to achieve the same level of performance.

The stretch-shortening cycle has a profound influence on the power output of explosive movements and on movement efficiency. These characteristics of the stretch-shortening cycle may be independent of strength levels in trained athletes, but they can be improved by training.[2] Therefore, athletes should incorporate specific training of the stretch-shortening cycle, also referred to as *plyometrics*, into their programs to maximize speed and agility. Think back to our boxer. If he could bring his arm back another inch, gain more stretch (like a rubber band), or load, to the muscles and deliver the punch in the same amount of time, the stored energy released would help increase the force of the punch delivered.

ANTHROPOMETRIC VARIABLES

Anthropometric variables, such as height, weight, body fat, and length and circumference of the limbs and trunk, may play a major role in athletic success. For example, a short person with a lower center of gravity and shorter limbs can conceivably change direction faster than a taller person with a higher center of gravity and longer limbs. Furthermore, assuming that two athletes weigh the same amount, it stands to reason that the leaner athlete would be able to produce greater force than the athlete with more body fat. This is because the fitter athlete has a greater amount of lean muscle mass.

In some sports, such as basketball, height may be an advantage, even though taller people change direction more slowly. A tall basketball player may be able to generate more force with his long lever arms. In contrast, a shorter wrestler's height may provide a distinct advantage since it allows him to change direction more quickly, due to his leverage and stability. Here, shorter lever arms and a lower center of gravity allow the wrestler to execute movements more quickly. However, the shorter wrestler may produce less force than one with longer lever arms.

Many studies have investigated anthropometry to determine its potential as a predictor of athletic performance in specific sports, such as gymnastics, volleyball, basketball, rock climbing, swimming, freestyle wrestling, and 10-pin bowling.[7, 12, 26, 44, 46, 50] These studies found that athletes who perform at high levels of competition in their respective sports fit a certain physical profile.

What if an athlete does not fit the profile for his particular sport? Although not all athletes may be the next all-pro player in their sport or receive a gold medal at the Olympics, they all have the ability to improve a variety of factors connected with agility and quickness. Muscle strength and power, improved rate of force development, reaction time, and improved technique are all components that directly affect overall agility and quickness. Athletes can improve these factors with proper training methods and techniques.

One study found that boys with a higher percent of body fat had poorer performances in the 40-yard (37 m) dash and in agility tests than their slimmer counterparts.[3] By simply changing one anthropometric variable, percent of body fat, athletes may improve their performance in the 40-yard dash and agility tests. If inflexibility in the hamstrings and hip flexors is hindering range of motion, then improving mobility in these muscles could positively affect performance. For this reason, coaches and athletes should identify deficient areas and modify practice and training for the greatest improvement on performance.

TECHNIQUE

Success in most sports depends on athletes' ability to rapidly and correctly initiate and stop movement in multiple directions while maintaining good body control and joint position. Athletes can change directions more effectively by ensuring the body is in the best possible position to produce, reduce, transfer, and stabilize both internal and external forces. If any segment of the body is out of position, athletes will not be able to achieve optimal agility performance. Thus, good technique is essential for maximizing agility performance and quickness.

Agility is a series of discrete tasks strung together to form what is called a *serial task*. Thus, the athlete must be able to combine the various movement patterns discussed in this section in the proper sequence and at the proper time while accelerating, decelerating, and transitioning in multiple directions. Therefore, athletes should first master individual movement patterns by practicing each of the skills in a controlled environment. Next, they may combine tasks and incorporate them into the specific movement patterns involved in a given sport. They can then use specific drills (see chapter 4 for examples) to improve footwork and speed in backward and lateral movements.

To produce the movement needed to change directions, athletes need to begin in good position. The universal athletic position (shown in figure 1.3) is a good beginning stance for a variety of movement patterns. Here, athletes slightly bend the knees and hips, slightly lean the torso forward, flatten the back, and position the head straight with eyes looking forward.[11] Other common positions include a staggered stance (see figure 1.4), such as the one used by defensive backs in football and a three-point stance (see figure 1.5) like defensive linemen use. Athletes can incorporate these stances to add greater sport specificity to a variety of multidirectional drills.

The same principles of position and body mechanics that are emphasized during power movements, such as doing explosive movements or linear speed work, are also critical when producing explosive directional changes. Thus, the propulsive forces generated through triple extension are vital for optimal agility performance. When backpedaling, athletes can achieve propulsion with the powerful action of the quadriceps and hip flexors (figure 1.6). The arm movement is similar to that used in forward sprinting.

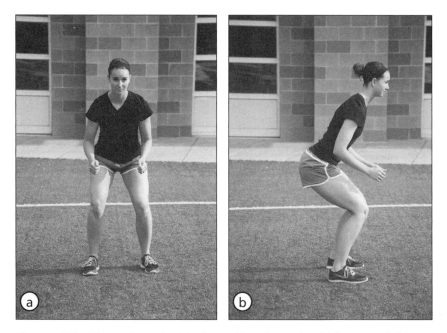

Figure 1.3 The universal athletic position from the *(a)* front and *(b)* side views.

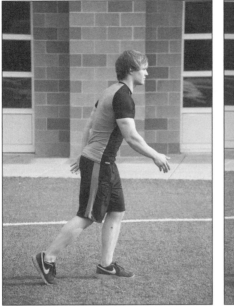

Figure 1.4   The staggered stance.

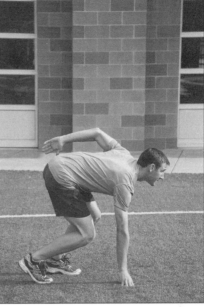

Figure 1.5   The three-point stance.

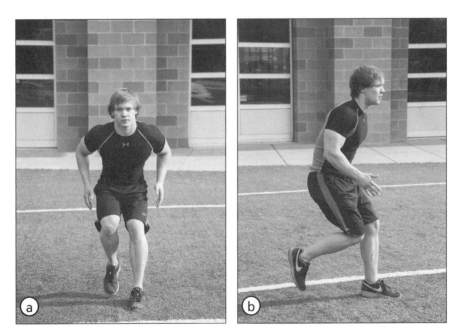

Figure 1.6   Proper body position for backpedaling from the *(a)* front and *(b)* side views.

In many cases, as athletes attempt to change direction, they pump their arms less, allowing the hands to cross the midline of the body or failing to swing the arms from the shoulders. Unfortunately, all of these extraneous movements may reduce their ability to produce quick directional changes. In order to produce force in any direction, athletes should use a proper arm swing that originates from the shoulder. Arms bent at approximately 90 degrees will help them produce greater force and more explosive movements.

The ability to reduce speed is also essential. Figure 1.7 shows the proper position for deceleration of a forward movement. Figure 1.8 on page 20

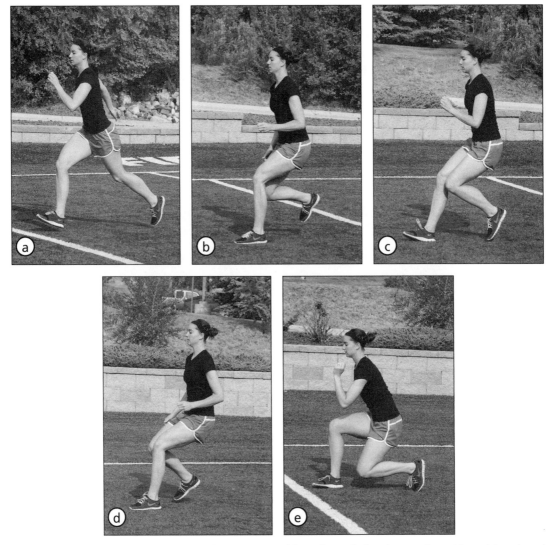

Figure 1.7 After the *(a)* last normal stride, the athlete *(b, c, d)* decelerates by taking abbreviated steps until she comes to a *(e)* full stop.

shows the proper position for both deceleration and acceleration of forward and lateral movements. These are the best possible positions for effectively producing and reducing speed. Notice during the forward movements (figure 1.7) that the majority of the athlete's weight is on the ball of the foot. During lateral movements, it is on the medial aspect of the foot (figure 1.8). To prepare for any directional change, the angles of the ankle and knee should be about or less than 90 degrees, and the hips and center of gravity should be in a low position. The foot of the outside leg should remain outside the center of mass and the lower leg should point roughly in the direction of the desired movement.

The transfer of forces relies on the ability to control the center of mass and center of gravity. As the center of gravity shifts away from the center of mass, it causes movement. Athletes with great agility can control their center of mass and position their bodies in an optimal manner to control their center of gravity. If the movement of the center of mass is excessive, causing the center of gravity to move too far outside the body, the athlete may lose balance or even fall. The ability to control center of gravity and center of mass allows athletes to transfer force and power more efficiently and to perform at higher levels.

Athletes can improve their ability to change directions with balance, body control, and minimal loss of speed by widening their base of support and lowering their center of gravity. Figure 1.9 on page 22 shows the correct position and an example of an incorrect body position during the breakdown of a lateral movement. In figure 1.9a, the athlete's weight is distributed evenly on the inside of the foot and the knee is lined up over the ankle. In figure 1.9b, the majority of the athlete's weight is on the outside of the foot, and the ankle and knee are in a compromised position over the outside. Furthermore, notice in figure 1.9a how the athlete's shin is roughly pointing in the direction of the desired movement. Compare this to figure 1.9b, in which the athlete's shin is pointing in the opposite direction of the desired movement. This angle is inappropriate for generating the power necessary for explosive changes of direction. Furthermore, it places the joints in a vulnerable position for injury.

When changing direction, some sort of rotation generally must occur to transition from one movement pattern to the next.[17] For example, when transitioning from a forward sprint in one direction to one in the opposite direction, many athletes begin by turning the head, immediately followed by the shoulders and the trunk. This creates a shift in the body's center of mass that allows the athlete to turn the pelvis and hips in the intended direction

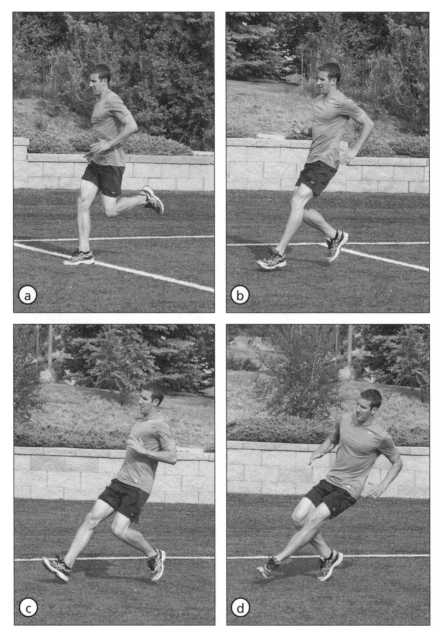

Figure 1.8 *(a, b, c)* The athlete decelerates by taking abbreviated steps and *(d)* turns laterally while lowering his center of gravity.

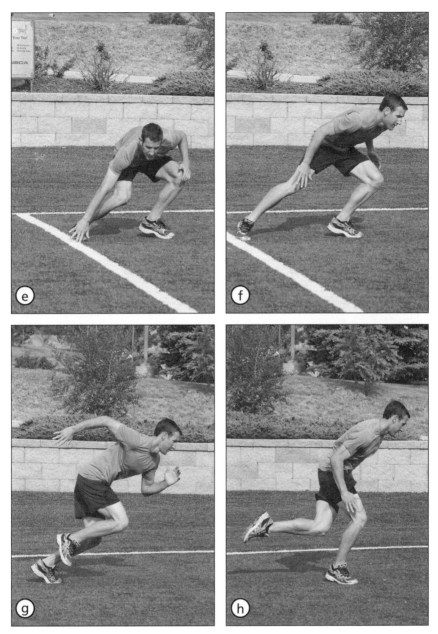

Figure 1.8 (continued) *(e, f)* While making a lateral change of direction, the athlete keeps the center of mass low and points the lower leg in the new direction. *(g, h)* The athlete then accelerates in the new direction.

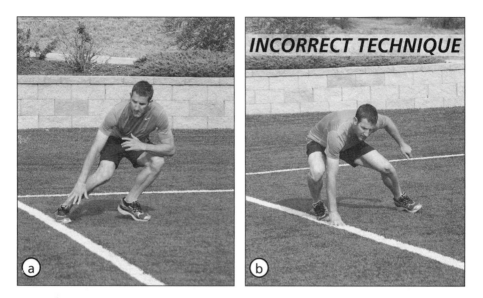

Figure 1.9 *(a)* The correct position for changing direction in lateral movement. *(b)* An incorrect body position is less effective and more likely to cause injury.

of movement.[17] Others initiate the rotation at the hip joint of the free leg, as shown in figure 1.10. The aim here is for the foot of the free leg to strike the ground on the next step, pointing in the intended direction for the next movement (see figure 1.11 on page 24). Many athletes attempt to initiate the rotation at the hip joint of the stance leg, transitioning the whole body in one fluid movement.

Regardless of the technique used, coaches should emphasize several specific cues to make certain the athlete is in the proper position to transition to the next movement with as little wasted motion as possible. Athletes should focus on punching the knees of the lead leg and pivoting the hips in the new direction. Correct body position produces power angles in the lower body. These help produce force and speed of movement. In order to make certain that they are fully turning their hips and generating maximal power, athletes should imagine that they have a camera at their navel. They should point the lens of the camera to take a picture of the direction they wish to go. Another cue for proper arm mechanics is to drive the lead elbow back in the direction of the planting foot to rotate the upper body and assist with core rotation. This action also helps athletes get into proper running form more efficiently.

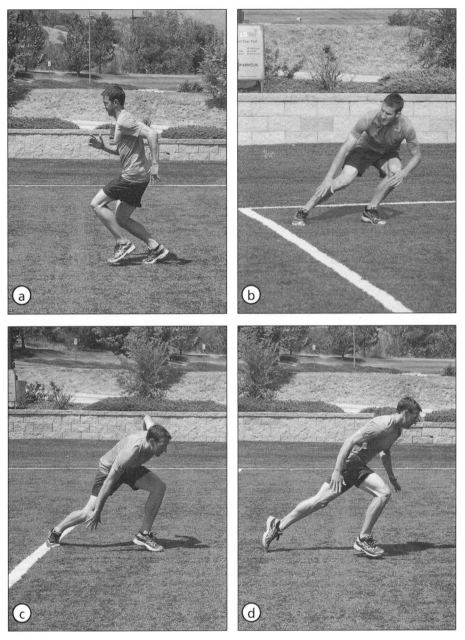

Figure 1.10 Transition movement with an open-leg knee drive. This change of direction skill teaches the ahtlete to plant and step as part of the change of direction motion. The athlete (a) begins to decelerate and (b) plants the outside leg, maintaining proper body position to load the muscles for the change of direction. The athlete (c) steps with the opposite leg, driving off the leg to propel in the new direction, and (d) sprints away.

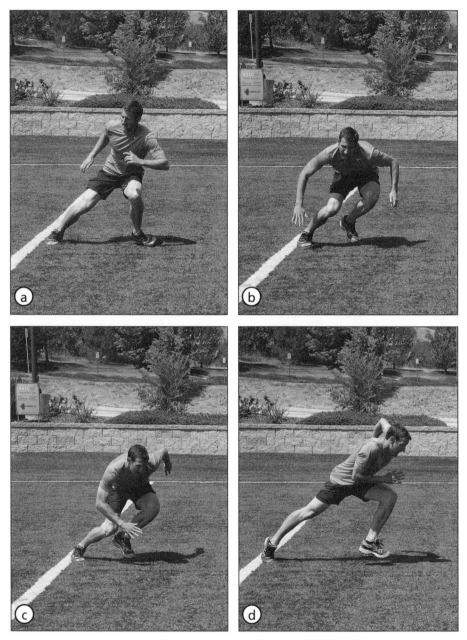

Figure 1.11 Transition movement with an opposite-leg knee drive. This change of direction skill teaches the athlete to push off as part of the change of direction motion. The athlete *(a)* lowers the center of gravity and loads the outside leg while opening the hips and *(b)* lifting the inside leg to change direction. The athlete *(c)* pushes off with the outside leg, turns hips, and gets ready to plant the inside foot with a positive shin angle to move in the opposite direction. The athlete *(d)* sprints away.

CHAPTER 2

Factors Determining Quickness

Jay Dawes
Jeremy Sheppard

The ability to identify relevant cues and execute the correct corresponding movements without delay largely determines an athlete's success.[9] If an athlete misreads or mistimes these cues, it can literally cost a goal, a game, or even a championship. Numerous perceptual and decision-making factors influence a player's reactive ability, or quickness, which also affects agility.

INFORMATION PROCESSING

Before athletes move, they must first identify the need to respond to a situation. They do this by collecting environmental cues from a variety of sensory input systems, such as the auditory, visual, and somatosensory systems.[18] For example, a running back waits for the quarterback to provide the auditory command to signal the start of a play. As he prepares to grab the handoff from the quarterback, he collects visual information about the position of the defense in an attempt to find a gap to run through. As would-be tacklers try to grab him, his somatosensory system gives his central nervous system feedback about the manual pressure the opponents are applying to his pads and body. Given this information, the player may be able to spin away from the attack. This scenario illustrates just one situation where environmental cues give athletes important information about their competitive environment.

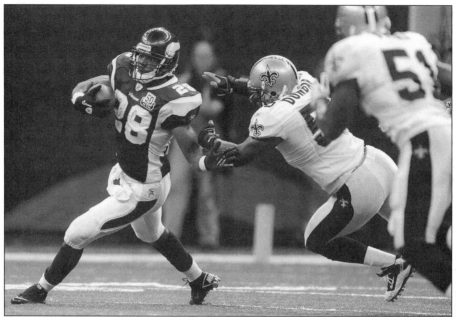

Running backs, such as Adrian Peterson, respond to a variety of environmental cues, allowing them to elude opponents.

The senses also collect information about specific patterns that indicate a particular type of play or an opponent's position. The athlete must interpret this information through perceptual skills to determine the appropriate response. Several variables affect the speed at which this information is processed, including stimulus clarity, intensity, mode, and experience.[17]

Stimulus clarity refers to the extent to which the stimulus is well defined and clear (i.e., in focus versus out of focus), and **stimulus intensity** deals with the strength or magnitude of the stimulus (loudness, brightness, and so on). The greater the clarity or intensity of an environmental stimulus, the faster the athlete will be able to process the information.[17]

The mode, or type of stimulus received also affects the speed at which it is detected. The time required to respond to a visual stimulus (approximately 180 to 200 milliseconds) is greater than the time required to respond to an auditory stimulus (approximately 140 to 160 milliseconds). Kinesthetic reaction time is the fastest (averaging 120 to 140 milliseconds).[22]

Finally, the athlete's level of experience has a profound effect on overall quickness. For example, athletes who are able to read or expect the next play based on their opponents' formation have a greater anticipatory advantage than those unable to identify these task-relevant cues. The ability to read the opposing player's actions is largely based on repetition and competitive experience over time.

Coaches should consider this information when developing open drills because it provides a better understanding of why athletes take longer to respond to some responses than others. (Open, or *reactive,* drills require athletes to respond to a stimulus to complete the drill.) For instance, this information shows that in most cases, an athlete will be able to respond to a sound more quickly than to a visual stimulus. Further, the type of stimulus the coach selects should be directly related to gamelike situations that the athlete may experience. For example, a sprinter should respond to a sound stimulus, since the same type of cue is used to initiate track events. In contrast, a sport-specific stimulus for a defensive lineman in football would involve movement, since football players look for visual stimuli in competition.

KNOWLEDGE OF SITUATIONS

The knowledge of specific sport situations helps players react more quickly to environmental cues. Cognitive research shows distinct differences between experts and nonexperts in visual search strategies.[1, 14, 16, 20, 21] This research indicates that expert performers use different cues than those with less experience do. For instance, an expert base runner may focus on a specific body movement by a pitcher (dipping the back leg, lifting the back foot off the pitching rubber, or lifting the front foot off the ground) to determine when he is going to make a delivery to the plate versus attempting a pickoff. Additionally, expert performers can find and focus in on relevant cues more quickly than their less experienced counterparts.[1, 23]

These differences between experts and nonexperts further emphasize the need for a highly specific training stimulus in order to improve reactive abilities. A generic stimulus, such as a light, is unlikely to be a valid measure for gauging performance. If expert performers utilize cues that are specific to tasks in a given sport domain, it seems unlikely that a generic stimulus would be ideal for improving recognition of a situation. In other words, a general reaction demand is unlikely to increase performance for a specific demand in a sport. In addition, it may not be a valid method for evaluating response-time differences between players of varying performance levels in the specific domain of their sport.[1, 14, 23]

Using the human model for information processing (see figure 2.1 on page 28), a given stimulus, prior to initiating a response, produces specific mental operations based on the subject's retrieval of stored information from memory. The accuracy and speed of this response depends on previously stored information that is specific to that situation.[8] If the stimulus used in training lacks specificity to the sport setting, then the training methods for decreasing response time are less valid and less likely to improve sport performance.

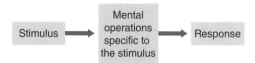

Figure 2.1 Information processing model.

Adapted from R.H. Cox, 2002, *Sport psychology: Concepts and applications*, 5th ed. (New York: McGraw-Hill), 133.

By collecting and processing information that occurs during sport performance, the athlete may begin to recognize specific types of patterns that indicate certain situations. For example, the trajectory or spin of a ball, the direction and speed of an opponent, or the opposition's position are all possible patterns that an experienced athlete may use to gain advantage over those with less experience. In many sports, the better an athlete is at recognizing and interpreting these patterns, the greater his potential for reacting quickly and accurately to the given stimulus.[17, 18] In a sport like American football, specific cues may alert the defense whether a passing or a running play is about to occur. If the defender is able to interpret these cues quickly, he is more likely to be in the correct position to make a necessary play.

This ability to recognize specific patterns is a skill that athletes can develop through experience and learning. Thus, both the amount and type of practice are important. As a player's knowledge of a particular situation increases and he becomes more familiar with the correct movement response in relation to the stimulus displayed, his reaction time or quickness will improve. For this reason, during the initial stages of learning, athletes should perform closed, preprogrammed agility drills for technique mastery. However, as

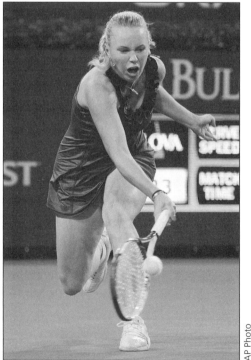

AP Photo

Knowledge of sport situations allows an experienced player, such as Caroline Wozniacki, to read a ball for a successful return.

they perfect technique and gain greater experience in their respective sports, open, unplanned quickness drills with appropriate cues may better improve their sport performance, due to greater specificity of training.

DECISION-MAKING SKILLS

Once the athlete has collected information about the environment and the situation, he must decide which actions or responses will yield the greatest success. Successful decision making requires both speed and precise movement. When the athlete has decided which specific movement to make based on information collected from the environment, a message is sent to the motor cortex to retrieve the desired movement pattern from memory. When it is received, the brain sends a message to the working skeletal muscles through the spinal cord to produce the desired movement.[22] If athletes choose the correct response, their opportunities for success increase exponentially. If they choose an incorrect movement, the result can be devastating.

The fake is a popular concept in many sports. In this type of play, an athlete indicates the initial stages of one movement and then quickly performs another movement to its completion. Players do this to give the opposition incorrect cues so that they cannot respond correctly or quickly enough to effectively defend the movement. If opposition players respond to the first (deceptive) movement, they will suffer a delay as they attempt to respond to the second (actual) movement. In the previous example, if the pitcher appears to be about to deliver the baseball to the plate but instead attempts a pickoff, this may cause the base runner a momentary delay, causing him to be picked off at the current base. If the runner attempts to steal, he may get caught in a rundown between bases.

The number of stimuli in the environment and the total number of possible actions largely determine the athlete's ability to select an appropriate response.[17, 18] Typically, reactions are classified as either *simple* or *choice*.[17] Simple reaction time refers to the presentation of a stimulus that has only one correct response, such as a gun being fired to signal the start of a footrace. Choice reactions require an athlete to select an appropriate response to one of several unanticipated stimuli.[18] Choice reaction time is important for sports that require athletes to respond to the movements of other players and to select appropriate responses based on these movements. These types of sports tend to be chaotic and unpredictable.[5] For example, as defenders in soccer follow their opponent dribbling downfield, they must watch their opponent's body position, offensive patterns of the opposition, and the location of their own teammates in order to take the most appropriate action and to best defend against the offensive attack.

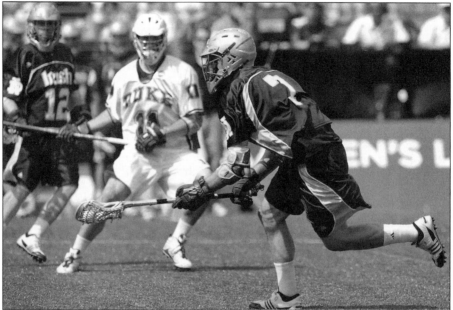

Mark Goldman/Icon SMI

Sports, such as lacrosse, create a chaotic environment in which players must react to multiple stimuli.

According to Hick's law, the amount of time required to prepare a response to a stimulus depends on the possible number of responses present.[17] Athletes can perform simple reaction tasks more quickly than choice reaction tasks because in those situations, only one stimulus is presented and only one correct response is possible. As the number of stimuli in the environment increases, the athlete has a greater number of alternative responses to select from in order to perform the correct motor task or skill. As a result, the amount of time required to execute a particular movement increases.[17]

Many experts believe simple reaction time is much harder, if not impossible, to alter through training because it is primarily related to genetics and the speed of the central nervous system. However, training and experience may significantly improve choice reaction time.[18] For this reason, athletes must incorporate some form of sport-specific reactive-agility training into their overall strength and conditioning programs to improve their ability to respond quickly to multiple stimuli in a chaotic sport environment.

ANTICIPATION

When athletes can accurately predict an event and organize their movements in advance, they can initiate an appropriate response more quickly than if they had waited to react to a stimulus. With experience, they gain greater knowledge of how long it takes to coordinate their own movements (known as *effector anticipation*) with certain environmental regularities and opponent tendencies in a given situation (*perceptual anticipation*). In addition, if athletes can predict which play will be used (*spatial anticipation*) and when it will occur (*temporal anticipation*), they will be able to form an appropriate response before the stimulus is presented.

Athletes who anticipate accurately can gain a large competitive advantage over their opposition. Anticipation is possible in nearly all sports. For example, by watching how an opponent pivots or drops the hips, a rugby player can get an idea of what direction an opponent is going or what movement he is trying to execute. When a pitcher throws a ball into the dirt, a base runner successfully steals a base due to the trajectory of the pitch as the ball was released.

Early studies involving anticipation and reaction time were based on generic stimuli and generic athletic responses.[7, 13] Some scientists have stressed that in order to truly assess and train the visual and recognition skills required in athletics, future research about anticipation and reaction time should involve a sport-specific presentation.[3] Experimental evidence demonstrated that generic visual-training approaches to motor learning are most likely ineffective because they train perceptual factors that do not influence performance in sports or gamelike situations. From these findings, the authors suggest that sport-specific protocols that utilize perceptual skills (such as pattern recognition and anticipation) may be best for establishing the appropriate context, or link, to skills in a particular sport.[3] High-performance athletes focus on anticipatory cues that are directly linked to specific signals displayed by their opponents.[1, 3, 11] Therefore, at this time, research provides compelling support for the use of sport-specific scenarios and stimuli in training programs.

As a component of perceptual and decision-making factors, anticipation appears to be a trainable quality, since athletes are able to improve these skills as they gain more competitive experiences.[2, 3, 10, 11, 19] Thus, this area of training is worthy of attention. When training anticipation skills, the primary goal should be to improve both the accuracy and the speed of responses.

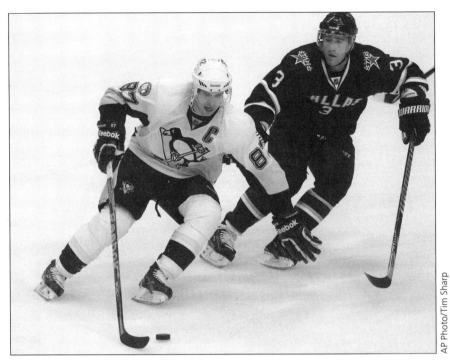

AP Photo/Tim Sharp

Through anticipatory cues an experienced hockey player, such as Sydney Crosby, can gain a competitive advantage over opponents.

For coaches, the previous findings in perceptual and decision-making research support using sport-specific scenarios. Scenarios that provide a stimulus relevant to the sporting environment may help athletes develop better anticipation skills through the refinement of search strategies, response speed and accuracy, pattern recognition, and decision-making abilities.

AROUSAL LEVEL

Arousal, or an athlete's overall level of central nervous system excitement and activation, plays a significant role in the ability to perform both quickly and accurately. The inverted *U* principle further explains the relationship between arousal and performance.[4, 18] Figure 2.2 shows the inverted *U* hypothesis, which states that arousal facilitates performance to a certain point. If the arousal level is too low or too high, the athlete fails to produce high-level performance.[18] The zone of optimal functioning, or simply *the zone,* is the level of arousal for the best integration of both the mental and physical processes associated with maximal performance.[12, 15] It is typified by several

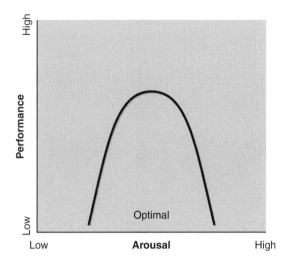

Figure 2.2 Inverted *U* principle.

Reprinted, by permission, from B.D. Hatfield and G.A. Walford, 1987, "Understanding anxiety: Implications for sport performance," *National Strength & Conditioning Association Journal* 9(2): 60-61.

factors, including improved automaticity (autopilot) and the increased ability to identify task-relevant cues and to ignore environmental cues that are irrelevant to performance.[18]

Typically, if athletes' arousal levels are too low, they may focus too much on irrelevant environmental cues. Since their environmental focus may be too broad, these perceptual distractions may not allow them to pick up on relevant environmental stimuli. Perceptual narrowing, or *tunnel vision,* may also occur as arousal levels continue to rise. This may hinder athletes' ability to identify task-relevant cues, thus increasing reaction time.

Ideally, athletes can identify the optimal level of arousal required to switch focus from broad to narrow. For example, when tennis players serve a ball, they initially have a broad focus as they scan the court to determine where they would like to hit the ball. They would then switch to a narrow focus during the serve. Once the serve is complete, they switch back to a broader focus to track their opponent and to anticipate where the opponent will return the ball. The server may be able to gain anticipatory clues from the position of the opponent's body or the position of the opponent's racquet when it strikes the ball. When the server sees the ball leave the opponent's racquet, he switches back to a narrower focus to concentrate on seeing the ball as it comes to his racquet, allowing for an effective reply.

For this reason, during practice, athletes may benefit from using open-skilled, or reactive, games that replicate situations that may be perceived as threatening. Examples include an opponent attempting to score a goal or a challenge that relates to performing a task more quickly than a competitor does. Drills that force players to perform in a competitive situation enhance their confidence and skill in adapting to new sport situations. This game-like environment allows players to adapt their skills and better control their arousal levels under the pressure of competition.

In conclusion, athletes' ability to achieve optimal agility and quickness performance depends largely on their perceptual and decision-making skills. In order to fully develop these capabilities, athletes must continue to gain experience identifying task-relevant cues in their respective sports by training in gamelike conditions and using sport-specific training cues and methods aimed at improving cognitive abilities and decision-making skills.

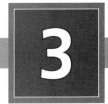

Testing Agility and Quickness

Jason Jones

Testing agility and quickness involves more than lining up a few cones and grabbing a stopwatch. A proper assessment for the specific demands, distances, and movements involved in a sport should provide valuable information for both the coach and athlete. Therefore, administrators should carefully select tests for athlete evaluation. Coaches and athletes can use the tests and evaluation drills featured in this chapter in several ways:

▶ *Predicting athletic potential.* Coaches often use field tests related to a given sport to predict an athlete's future ability to successfully perform a specific activity or sport.[1, 3, 5] Thus, the tests selected to assess athletic potential should mimic the specific movement patterns, muscle groups, and energy systems required for a particular sport in order to provide meaningful information and feedback.

▶ *Identifying strengths and weaknesses.* By determining which change-of-direction factors and perceptual and decision-making skills need improvement, the coach can make better choices about which drills should take priority in the athlete's training program. Further, periodic testing may give athletes, coaches, and trainers valuable information as to how effective an implemented training program has been.

▶ *Comparing athletes' performance levels.* Collecting testing data can help athletes gain a better understanding of how their performance levels compare with those of others. Coaches often use collected data to compare athletic performance, evaluate their programs, and track progress from one testing period to another and from season to season.

▶ *Improving motivation and goal setting.* Testing can help the coach and athlete set specific, measureable, and realistic goals to improve performance. Testing athletes regularly provides the coach and athlete with valuable information needed to create and modify the training program to meet specific goals.[1]

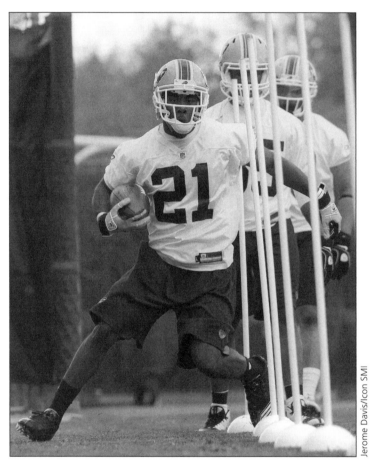

Jerome Davis/Icon SMI

Just as NFL teams use testing to evaluate players, coaches and athletes at all levels can use testing to predict and improve performance.

TEST SELECTION

When selecting a test to predict athletic performance, coaches must consider the validity, reliability, and objectivity of the assessment method. Choosing tests with these qualities can help a program succeed. Coaches should also make sure the proper tests are being done and should track the outcome of every testing session to see if the same parameters are being measured.

Validity

Validity refers to the degree that a test assesses what it intends or claims to measure.[2] For instance, power production is critical for success in sporting events that require jumping, sprinting, throwing, and striking. A successful vertical jump requires an athlete to explosively propel the body upward, working a variety of body segments in unison, especially the legs, hips, and trunk. Thus, coaches, trainers, and researchers often select this skill when assessing anaerobic power of the lower body.[4] Sports like basketball, volleyball, and football often utilize the vertical jump to predict performance.

Reliability

Reliability refers to the repeatability or consistency of a test.[2] If a test is truly reliable, the results should not greatly differ when multiple trials are performed. Several factors may influence the reliability of a test:

- ▶ Testing surface
- ▶ Clarity of instruction
- ▶ Experience of test administrator
- ▶ Number of trials and practice trials allowed
- ▶ Rest periods between tests
- ▶ Ambient temperature
- ▶ Time of day
- ▶ Motivational factors (i.e., spectators, tester, and teammate encouragement)
- ▶ Nutritional and hydration status
- ▶ Fatigue level

In order for a test to be valid, it must be reliable. However, reliability does not ensure that a test is valid. For example, an assessment of body mass index may be reliable, but the results may not be as accurate for those who are more athletic or muscular.

Objectivity

Objectivity is a form of reliability that refers to how the administrator collects test data.[2] Objectivity depends on several factors, such as the following:

▶ The administrators' experience and competence in administering the test

▶ Inter-rater reliability, or whether multiple testers are able to attain the same results

▶ Whether standardized testing procedures are followed to ensure that all athletes being tested receive consistent instructions and methods

High objectivity occurs when personal bias is alleviated. Multiple administrators should be able to give the same instructions for a test and obtain similar results.

TESTING PROCESS

In order to ensure consistent and accurate results, coaches must take certain steps to ensure proper data collection. Establishing protocol before testing begins is critical. Everyone involved in the testing process must understand what is expected of them as well as the specific methods and procedures to be used. When developing a testing protocol, address the items from the following section prior to assessment.

Sequence

After choosing valid, objective, and reliable tests, the administrator must decide the testing order. With proper order of testing, the coach can make sure to gather accurate data. Things to consider when choosing the testing order include the following:

▶ *Energy demands of the test.* Tests involving a display of power should be performed before endurance-type tests. Short-duration tests should be administered before longer-duration tests. For example, administrators should conduct an agility test prior to a test used to determine aerobic capacity, such as the 1.5-mile (2.4 km) running test, since fatigue from the aerobic test may negatively influence agility performance. Testing the energy systems at the right time offers the best results and gives the coach a better indication of athletes' status in terms of performance improvement.

▶ *Number of trials given for each test.* Often, multiple trials are a detriment to testing athletes because they do not have enough time for proper rest and recovery. If athletes perform a test while fatigued, they will likely not perform as well as they possibly can. This habit also increases the risk of injury. In general, it is good to offer three practice trials at a submaximal speed to allow the athlete to become familiarized with each test.

▶ *Number of athletes participating.* In order to maximize the flow of testing, the test administrator must organize the testing protocol to ensure athletes can complete all their testing in the allotted amount of time.

▶ *Number of testing administrators.* Depending on the number of athletes who are testing, it may be advantageous to have more than one test administrator to help maintain accurate and consistent records and execute testing protocols as intended. For example, in large groups, having at least one administrator to ensure that testing protocol is followed accurately and another to time and record scores makes the process much more manageable.

▶ *Equipment needed for each test.* Making sure that all assessment materials are available and ready for the day of testing is paramount for executing an efficient session. Coaches can create a quick checklist to better organize this process.

▶ *Recovery time.* In order to attain the best score possible on each measure, coaches should allow at least three to five minutes between trials. This reduces the negative effect of fatigue on the athletes and allows their ATP-CP energy systems to fully recover, ensuring that their technique does not suffer and that they have enough energy to give their best effort.

Equipment

In addition to administrative supplies, such as pencils, clipboards, and forms for recording results, the coach must also secure any equipment and safety supplies deemed necessary for the testing, including cones, stopwatches, a laser timing device, or a first-aid kit.

Environment

To ensure safe and accurate testing, the coach must confirm that the area used for testing is appropriate. The coach must make sure that the athlete is able to safely and effectively perform each test at maximal effort. The following are just a few questions that the athlete and coach should evaluate:

▶ Is the testing area free of any potential hazards or clutter?

▶ Is the athlete's footwear appropriate? Do the athletic shoes offer good support? If testing outdoors, would cleats are more appropriate?

▶ Is the athlete wearing athletic attire that will not restrict the ability to move freely (i.e., athletic shorts, or sweats)?

▸ Is the testing surface resilient and nonslip?

▸ Is the area large enough to allow athletes plenty of room to safely perform the test?

Staff

Typically, a coach serves as the testing supervisor. This entails overseeing the testing procedures, making sure that the process flows well, and obtaining accurate results. If multiple tests will be performed, the coach may want to get additional administrative support for data collection. The support staff must be educated on the proper rules and test setup, as well as on any motivational instructions. Since motivation plays a large role in the results of physical tests, it is the coach's responsibility to establish the following:

▸ Whether spectators or other athletes will be allowed to offer verbal support for the athlete being tested

▸ Whether the athlete will receive immediate feedback about the performance (i.e., corrections, knowledge of results)

▸ Whether athletes will be allowed to view others' results

▸ Whether the results will determine which athletes will make the team, and whether the athletes will have this knowledge

Administration

Prior to testing day, the lead testing administrator should meet with the other administrators to practice giving the selected tests and to clarify any procedural questions. Administrators should read and study all testing instructions and should practice each test numerous times to ensure familiarity. The chief testing administrator should also discuss data collection to ensure uniformity of results. Since each test involves some instruction, the chief administrator must also decide how many practice trials the athlete will be allowed and how each test will be scored. For instance, will the athletes be evaluated on their best score or will the average of several scores be used?

Customization

In some situations, coaches may select certain protocols to obtain a better assessment of the movement done for a specific sport. For example, the pro-agility test is commonly used by football coaches and athletes. As a result, many of the standards and norms established for this test are based on the athlete starting in a three-point stance. Athletes from sports that do not require this stance may prefer a two-point stance. However, both the testing administrator and those being tested must understand that while they will be able to compare their pre- and post-test scores to one another, the established norms that use the three-point stance will not apply because of the difference in testing protocol.

AGILITY AND QUICKNESS TESTS

Administrators may use the tests on pages 42 to 53 to determine an athlete's current level of agility and quickness, identify areas for improvement, and gauge the effectiveness of an agility training program. Table 3.1 provides an overview of the tests included in this chapter.

Table 3.1 Agility and Quickness Tests

Test name	Tests agility	Tests quickness	Page number
Box step-off landing assessment*			42–43
Illinois agility test	x		44–45
5-0-5 agility test	x		46
Pro-agility shuttle	x		47
Three-cone shuttle test	x		48
Four corners test	x		49
Hexagon test	x	x	50
Quadrant jump test	x	x	51
T test	x		52
J.P. shuttle (60-yard shuttle)	x		53

*This test does not test agility or quickness. It is a qualitative movement screen that also tests eccentric strength.

BOX STEP-OFF LANDING ASSESSMENT

Purpose

To determine an athlete's readiness before beginning a program in agility and quickness

Application

This test examines the ability to maintain stability and handle additional stress that comes from jumping, bounding, and deceleration. It is also good for use with beginning athletes.

Equipment

6- to 18-inch (15–46 cm) plyometric box

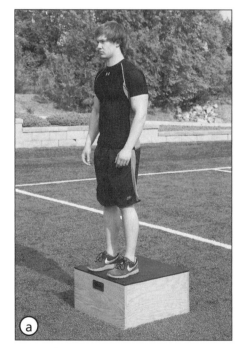

Starting position.

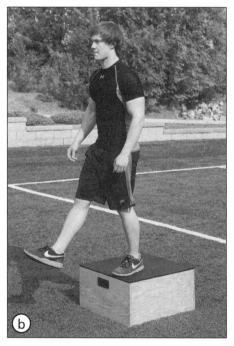

Stepping.

Procedure

The athlete stands on a plyometric box that is 6 to 18 inches (15–46 cm) high and assumes a comfortable, upright stance with feet shoulder-width apart. He should step from the box, landing on the floor in an athletic position with even pressure on both feet and then in a controlled manner perform a bodyweight squat. The athlete should maintain proper body alignment (chest up, shoulders back, feet approximately shoulder-width apart, and knees in alignment with toes) and should land in a balanced position.

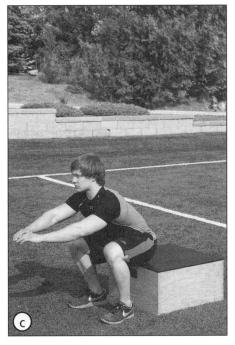

Squatting position.

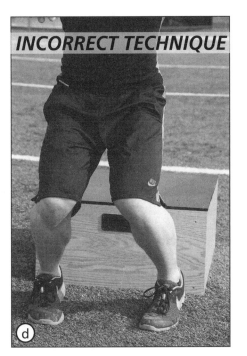

INCORRECT TECHNIQUE

Incorrect landing position.

ILLINOIS AGILITY TEST

Purpose

To assess technique and speed during straight sprinting and changes in direction

Application

For sports that require a change of direction out of linear movement, this test helps assess athletes' ability to cut and efficiently change direction. Examples include a receiver in American football running a pass route or a soccer player dribbling the ball and moving around defenders.

Equipment

Laser timing device or stopwatch, measuring tape, 8 cones or markers, and a flat, nonslip surface

Testing Layout

Set up four cones in a rectangle 10 meters (10.9 yd) long and 5 meters (5.5 yd) wide. The two cones at one end (A and D) mark the start and finish of the test. Cones B and C are at the other end. Place the remaining four cones (numbered 1 through 4) down the center of the testing area 3 meters apart.

Procedure

The athlete should begin by lying on the belly with hands flat on the floor, elbows up in the air, and head facing the starting line at cone A. On the *go* signal, the athlete gets up as quickly as possible and sprints 10 meters (10.9 yd) to cone B. The administrator starts the timing device when the athlete first moves. The athlete then sprints to cone 1 in the center of the testing area, weaves in and out of cones 1 through 4 using a zigzag motion, circles cone 4, and then returns to cone 1, weaving through the center cones in the opposite direction. After turning around cone 1, the athlete sprints 10 meters (10.9 yd) to cone C and then back across the starting line between cones A and D. The administrator stops the timing device when the athlete reaches cone D. Table 3.2 provides general standards and norms for this test.

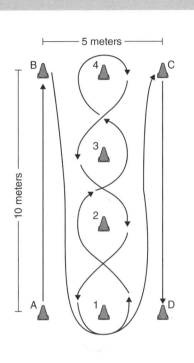

Table 3.2 Illinois Agility Test Norms

			Rating		
	Excellent	**Good**	**Average**	**Fair**	**Poor**
Males	<15.2	16.1–15.2	18.1–16.2	18.3–18.2	>18.3
Females	<17.0	17.9–17.0	21.7–18.0	23.0–21.8	>23.0

Adapted, by permission, from M. Roozen, 2004, "Action-reaction: Illinois Agility Test," *NSCA's Performance Training Journal* 3(5): 5-6.

5-0-5 AGILITY TEST

Purpose

To test technique, strength during acceleration and deceleration, and change-of-direction speed

Application

This test is good for athletes who want to gain maximum acceleration, not just top-end speed. This skill is essential for certain sport actions, such as a baseball or softball player stealing second base. The key here is acceleration, because the athlete will not reach top speed before needing to decelerate at second base or into a slide.

Equipment

Laser timer or stopwatch, nonslip running surface, and 6 cones or markers

Testing Layout

Establish a starting line by placing two cones 2 to 3 meters (2.2 to 3.3 yd) apart. Place two more cones 10 meters (10.9 yd) from the starting line and position a laser timer or a person with a stopwatch there (timing line). Place a third pair of cones (turning line) 15 meters (16.4 yd) from the starting line.

Procedure

When ready, the athlete begins this test using a flying start, sprinting from the starting line toward the 15-meter (16.4 yd) line. The athlete stops and turns there, and then heads back toward the starting line, running through the 10-meter (10.9 yd) line and continuing to accelerate past the starting line. The test administrator starts the timer when the athlete first breaks the plane of the 10-meter (10.9 yd) line (timing line) and stops the timer when he returns past the same mark. The administrator records the best result of three trials. A variation of this test is to have the athlete change direction with both the right and left legs and to record the best of three trials for each leg.

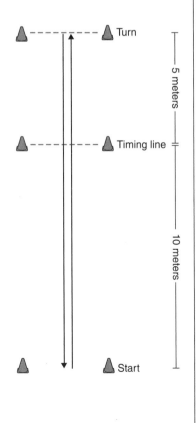

PRO-AGILITY SHUTTLE

Purpose

To assess technique while performing multiple changes of direction, leg strength, and power

Application

Because of the constant changes of direction needed, this test applies to nearly all power sports. It tests proper body positions and mechanics and measures the ability to start, accelerate, and decelerate.

Equipment

A laser timing device or stopwatch, measuring tape or marked field, 3 cones or markers, and a flat, nonslip surface

Testing Layout

Set up three cones 5 yards (4.6 m) apart to form a straight line that covers a total distance of 10 yards (9.1 m).

Procedure

The athlete begins facing the middle cone (cone 1) and puts one hand on the ground to assume a three-point stance. On command, the athlete turns to the right and runs 5 yards to cone 2, then touches the ground next to it with the right hand. The athlete then turns and sprints 10 yards to cone 3, then touches the ground next to it with the left hand. Finally, the athlete turns and finishes by sprinting back to and through the starting area (cone 1). Timing begins as soon as the athlete moves out of the three-point stance and stops when the athlete passes through the finish line. The administrator should record the best time out of three trials.

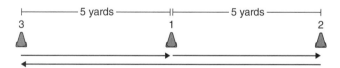

THREE-CONE SHUTTLE TEST

Purpose

To assess technique, acceleration, and change-of-direction speed

Application

Like the pro-agility shuttle, this test applies to skills used in most power sports, including body position and proper technique of movement, starting, acceleration, deceleration, and change of direction.

Equipment

A laser timing device or stopwatch, measuring tape or marked field, 3 cones or markers, and a flat, nonslip surface

Testing Layout

Place three cones in an *L* pattern with legs of equal length. The end cones are 1 and 3 and the one at the 90-degree corner is cone 2. Cones 1 and 2 and cones 2 and 3 are positioned 5 yards (4.6 m) apart.

Procedure

The athlete starts in a sport-specific stance next to cone 1 and faces cone 2. On command, the athlete sprints to cone 2 (see figure a), bends down, and touches the ground with the right hand. The athlete turns 180 degrees and sprints back to cone 1, bends down, and touches the ground with the right hand again. He then sprints back to cone 2 (see figure b), turns around it on the outside, and sprints to cone 3. At cone 3, the athlete turns around it on the outside and sprints back to cone 2. At cone 2, he plants the feet, turns left, and sprints back to cone 1 to finish the test. Timing starts on the command and stops when the athlete returns to cone 1.

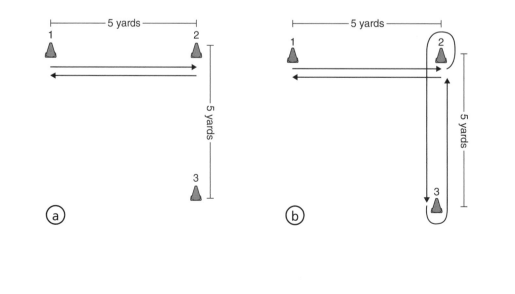

FOUR CORNERS TEST

Purpose

To assess movement skills and change-of-direction speed while moving forward, side to side, and backward

Application

Athletes frequently need to move forward, laterally, and backward. In many sports, such as basketball, athletes must be able to move in one direction, decelerate, stop, and then move in another direction as quickly as possible. This test provides a good indication of how well athletes move in multiple directions for their sport.

Equipment

A laser timing device or stopwatch, measuring tape, 4 cones or markers, and a flat, non-slip surface

Testing Layout

Position four cones to form a 10-yard (9.1 m) square.

Procedure

The athlete starts in a three-point stance next to cone 1 and faces cone 2. On the *go* command, the athlete sprints to and around cone 2 on the outside. Then, while continuing to face the same direction, the athlete shuffles sideways to the outside of cone 3. From cone 3, the athlete backpedals as fast as possible to cone 4, and then finishes by turning left and sprinting past cone 1. Timing starts on the command and stops when the athlete moves past cone 1 after completing the square. The athlete must move around the outside of each cone for a successful test.

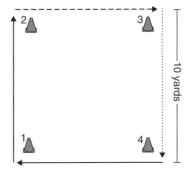

HEXAGON TEST

Purpose

To test body control and the ability to adjust strides for acceleration and deceleration

Application

This test helps measure body control with high force production, and how well athletes can not only accelerate and get to a new position, but also control body segments, decelerate, and move in another direction without losing form and control. For example, in basketball or soccer, defensive players must react to outside stimuli (another player or the movement of a ball) and adjust their positions accordingly or adjust how they defend an opponent.

Equipment

Measuring tape, chalk or tape for marking ground, a stopwatch, and an appropriate surface for jumping

Testing Layout

Using athletic tape or chalk, make a hexagon on the ground or floor. Each side of the hexagon should be 2 feet (60.5 cm) in length and each angle should be 120 degrees. Designate the sides as 1 through 6.

Procedure

The athlete starts by standing in the middle of the hexagon. On the *go* signal, the athlete hops over line 1 with both feet and then hops back into the middle of the hexagon in the same manner. The athlete repeats this process, hopping over each line in order (1 through 6) and back to the center of the hexagon pattern for three full revolutions. For all the hops, the athlete should face in the original direction. Timing starts on the signal and stops at the end of the third round when the athlete comes back to the center. This test should be performed both clockwise and counterclockwise.

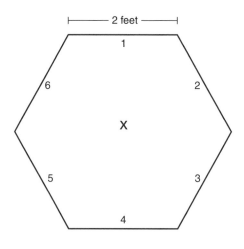

QUADRANT JUMP TEST

Purpose

To test body control and the ability to adjust strides for acceleration and deceleration

Application

This test is great for any sport that requires multiple changes of direction.

Equipment

Tape measure, chalk or tape for marking ground, and a stopwatch

Testing Layout

Mark a cross pattern on the floor. Number the resulting quadrants 1 through 4 as follows: The first quadrant is on the bottom left, the second on the upper left, the third on the top right, and the fourth on the bottom right.

Procedure

The athlete stands in the middle of the cross in a good power position with both feet about shoulder-width apart and faces into quadrant 1. On the *go* command, the administrator starts timing, and the athlete jumps forward into quadrant 1. Then, in sequence, he continues jumping into each quadrant as fast as possible with control, facing the same direction throughout the test. The pattern continues as rapidly as possible for 10 seconds when time is called. During the 10 seconds, the test administrator counts the number of jumps and assesses the quality of each jump. Each jump in which the athlete lands with both feet entirely within the correct quadrant earns one point. Jumps in which the athlete touches a line or lands with one or both feet in an incorrect quadrant result in a half-point penalty. After a three-minute rest, the athlete repeats the test. The administrator records the best score. When available, an additional administrator should assist so that one person times the test and the other scores the test.

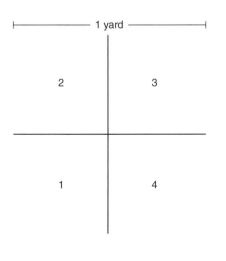

T TEST

Purpose

To test the ability to adjust strides for acceleration and deceleration, change-of-direction speed, and body control while moving forward, backward, and laterally

Application

This test looks at acceleration patterns and mimics the movements of most power sports and the quick directional changes needed in small spaces, such as in volleyball.

Equipment

A laser timing device or stopwatch, measuring tape, 4 cones or markers, and a flat, nonslip surface

Testing Layout

Set out four cones in a *T* pattern. Cone 1 is the bottom of the *T* and serves as the starting line. Cone 2 is placed 10 yards (9.1 m) from cone 1. It is the middle of the top of the *T*. Form the rest of the top by placing cones 5 yards (4.6 m) to the left (cone 3) and right (cone 4) of cone 2.

Procedure

The athlete begins at cone 1 in a stance appropriate for his sport. A football lineman might begin in a three-point stance, and a basketball player would start in a good athletic position. The athlete should use the same starting position for each trial. On the *go* command, the athlete sprints to cone 2 and touches the top of the cone with the right hand. The athlete then side shuffles to cone 3 without crossing the feet. The athlete touches the top of cone 3 with the left hand. The athlete then shuffles sideways to cone 4 and touches its top with the right hand. Next, the athlete shuffles back to cone 2, touching it with the left hand. The athlete then plants and backpedals to cone 1 through the starting line. Timing starts on the command and stops as the athlete passes through the starting line.

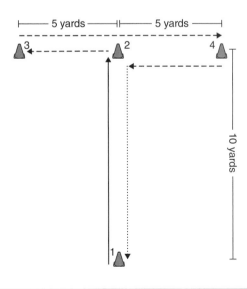

J.P. SHUTTLE (60-YARD SHUTTLE)

Purpose

To test body lean and posture, straight-sprinting speed, muscle qualities, and the abilities to adjust strides for acceleration and deceleration and to change direction using different flying-start distances

Application

This test not only tests acceleration and deceleration in the first few seconds of movement, but also looks at athletes' ability to use quickness and agility skills over time. It provides information about different segments of agility and quickness to help coaches create a training program that works on the start of a movement or parts of deceleration while examining body position and body control.

Equipment

A laser timing device or stopwatch, measuring tape, 5 cones or markers, and a flat, nonslip surface

Testing Layout

Place five cones in a straight line, spacing them 5 yards (4.6 m) apart. The center cone, labeled number 1, serves as the starting line. The cones to the right of the center cone are numbered 2 and 4, and the cones to the left are numbered 3 and 5.

Procedure

The athlete faces the center cone and straddles the starting line. On the *go* command, the athlete sprints to cone 2, touches it with the left hand, then sprints to cone 3 and touches it with the right hand. The athlete then sprints to cone 4, touching it with the left hand, and then sprints back to cone 5, touching it with the right hand. Finally, the athlete sprints back to the original starting line (at cone 1). Timing starts on the command and stops when the athlete reaches cone 1 for the final time. The test should be repeated after a five-minute rest. The administrator records the best time for the runs.

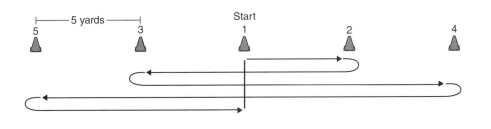

CHAPTER 4

Agility Drills

Mark Roozen
Mike Nitka
David Sandler

As chapter 1 discusses, proper footwork and good technique are critical for changing direction with skill and precision. This chapter provides numerous agility drills that focus on the speed and technique of changing direction. It also offers suggestions on how to modify each of these preprogrammed (closed) training drills to create semicontrolled (open) training drills that require both preprogrammed and reactive components.

Not every drill is appropriate or should be used for all athletes. Coaches should examine each drill to see where it fits with the level of specific athletes. Using proper progression is important when implementing any training element into a program, and the same is true with agility drills. Proper progression follows these guidelines:

▶ *Level 1 (basic) agility* focuses on technique and body position. This level uses basic cuts and movement patterns.

▶ *Level 2 (intermediate) agility* combines more complex movement patterns and involves transitional movements, good body mechanics and position, and change-of-direction speed that require higher levels of force and power.

▶ *Level 3 (advanced) agility* uses skills and drills that mimic real game or competitive situations. (Chapter 5 presents level 3 drills.)

The level used depends on the athlete's skill. Full recovery is needed to improve agility. During drills, if technique, speed of movement, or the ability to maintain high performance levels decreases, then athletes are working on conditioning rather than on the qualities needed to improve agility. Coaches should follow proper training guidelines for rest and recovery for their class of athletes. Implementing a systemic approach and following proper progression will greatly improve athletes' performance levels.

PREDRILL DYNAMIC WARM-UP

Athletes should warm up before performing any type of agility training. Proper warm-up increases blood flow to the muscles and neurological activity and gives the athlete time to mentally prepare for the workout. One of the most effective ways to prepare the body for physical activity is to perform dynamic warm-up activities. Furthermore, this type of movement preparation may help reduce the risk of some types of injuries. The following are just a few drills that can be performed as a dynamic warm-up.

Stationary Arm Warm-Up

The athlete sits with legs out in front, heels touching the ground, knees slightly bent, arms at the side, and elbows bent at a 90-degree angle. (The exercise may also be performed in a standing position.) She begins by moving one arm forward and the other backward so that one hand is at eye level and the opposite hand is level with the back hip pocket. Then, she moves the front arm to the back and the back arm to the front. She should start off at about half speed, then increase speed when she has achieved proper technique and form. At any point, if the athlete breaks technique or form, the coach should stop the warm-up. The athlete builds up speed for 12 to 15 seconds or until she breaks form. The coach may repeat as desired with proper breaks between sets for full recovery. This dynamic warm-up can also serve as a technique drill for learning or reinforcing proper arm mechanics during running.

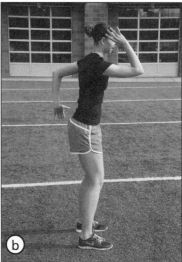

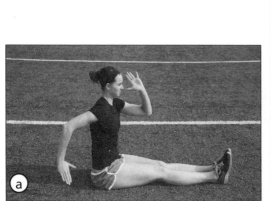

Sitting version.

Standing version.

Leg Swings Front to Back

The athlete stands perpendicular to a wall, fully extends the arm closest to the wall, and places the palm of the hand against it for support. She swings the leg closest to the wall forward and backward as quickly as possible with control. The athlete should perform 10 to 15 repetitions, and then turn to face the other direction and repeat with the other leg.

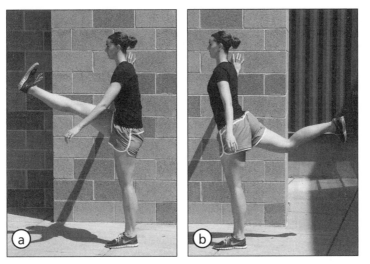

Forward swing.   Backward swing.

Leg Swings Side to Side

The athlete faces a wall, fully extending both arms to shoulder height and placing both palms against the wall for support. She lifts one leg and swings it from side to side across the body as quickly as possible with control. The athlete should perform 10 to 15 repetitions on each leg.

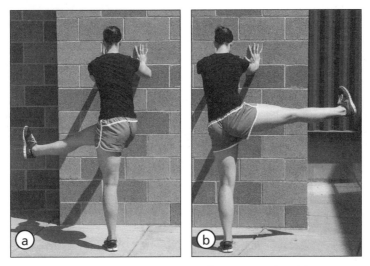

Swing across.   Swing out to the side.

Walking High-Knee Pulls

The athlete begins by flexing one hip and lifting the knee on that side as high as possible. Then, the athlete grabs the leg just below the knee with both hands and pulls the knee to the chest, keeping the back and chest up. The athlete returns the raised leg to the ground and repeats the action with the other leg. The exercise is continued by alternating legs with each step as the athlete walks forward for 10 yards (9 m).

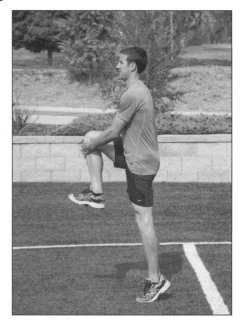

Lunge Walk With Twist

The athlete extends the arms directly in front of the chest at approximately shoulder level. She takes an exaggerated step forward, striking the ground with the heel first. Once the foot makes contact with the ground, the athlete flexes the knee of the lead leg until the top of the thigh is approximately parallel with the ground. She then rotates the hips and shoulders as far as possible toward the lead leg. If possible, the athlete should keep the arms extended. If needed, she can slightly bend the elbows for better balance and control. The knee of the lead leg should not move forward past the toes on that side. Also, the knee of the trail leg should not make contact with the ground. The athlete

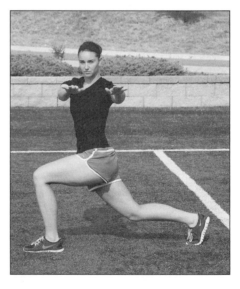

returns to the starting position by stepping forward with the trail leg, and then repeats the exercise, leading with the opposite leg. The athlete performs this drill for 10 yards (9 m), alternating the lead leg with each step.

Lateral Lunge Walk

The athlete extends the arms directly in front of the chest at approximately shoulder level. He takes an exaggerated step to the side. Once the foot touches the ground, the athlete bends the knee of the lead leg and lowers the body until the top of the thigh is approximately parallel with the ground. The arms remain extended throughout the duration of this exercise to assist with balance. The knee of the lead leg should not move forward past the toes. The trail leg should remain straight, but should not become locked. Those with limited flexibility might perform the movement with a slight bend in the knee. This drill is performed for 10 yards (9 m).

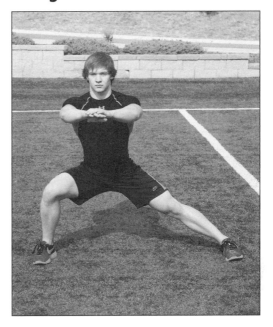

Toy Soldiers

While walking forward, the athlete swings one leg forward as high as possible, keeping it straight. She reaches the opposite arm out in front at about shoulder height and uses it as an anatomical landmark or target for the swinging foot. The other arm will rotate back behind the body to counteract the movement and to help control balance. The athlete continues walking forward, swinging and extending the opposite leg and arm. She performs the drill for 10 yards (9 m), alternating arms and legs with each step.

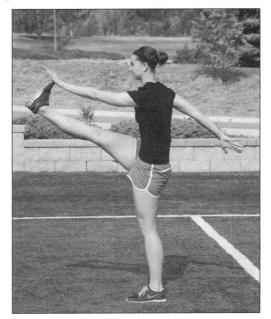

Butt Kicks

The athlete jogs forward and forcefully kicks the heels toward the buttocks with each stride. The heel of each foot should strike the rear end on that side. The knee of the kicking leg should stay in line with the stationary leg. The athlete should be careful not to let it swing back past the hip. This exercise is performed for 10 yards (9 m).

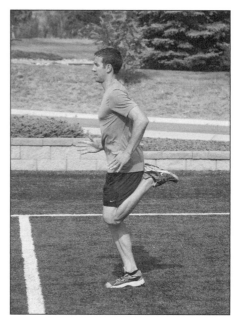

High-Knee Runs

The athlete runs forward, lifting the knee up as high as possible as each leg comes to the front. He should focus on pulling the toe up toward the shin and lifting the heel on the lead leg as he drives it toward the chest. This drill is performed for 10 yards (9 m).

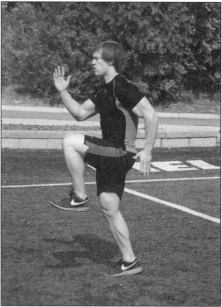

Quick Sprints

Quick sprints are a great finish to the dynamic warm-up because they prepare the body for faster, more vigorous movements. Quick sprints should be done on a field or area approximately 25 to 50 yards (23–46 m) in length in order to allow adequate space for accelerating and decelerating the body. The athlete begins by sprinting 10 to 25 yards (9–23 m) and then jogging for the remaining 10 to 25 yards. This routine is repeated two to four times.

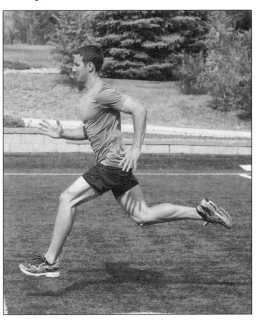

LINE DRILLS

Line drills are commonly used by coaches and athletes to improve footwork, speed, and coordination. Line drills are excellent for beginners since they are simple and require limited equipment. In fact, all that is needed is a boundary line (made from paint, chalk, or tape) on a gym floor, a sports field, or another nonslip, resilient surface. Athletes can vary the difficulty of line drills by altering combinations of upper- and lower-body movements and changing the complexity of footwork. (See chapter 6 for information about duration and number of repetitions.) The following are examples of line drills and their variations.

Forward and Backward Line Hops

LEVEL 1

The athlete stands parallel with the line and then hops back and forth over it with the feet together for a specified time period or number of repetitions. After the athlete lands for each hop, he should immediately push off again and hop to the other side of the line. No extra hops or bounces should occur.

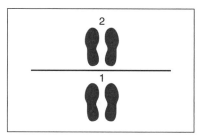

Single-Leg Variation

Hopping back and forth over the line can also be performed on one leg. The athlete should complete the drill for a specified time period or number of repetitions. The drill should be performed equally on each leg to ensure balanced training.

Lateral Line Hops

LEVEL 1

The athlete stands perpendicular with the line and then hops side to side over it for a specified time period or number of repetitions.

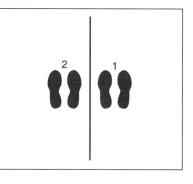

Single-Leg Variation

Hopping side to side over the line can also be performed on one leg. The athlete should complete the drill for a specified time period or number of repetitions. This drill should be performed equally on each leg to ensure balanced training.

Scissors

LEVEL 1

The athlete stands parallel with the line and then steps across with the right foot, straddling the line with the left foot behind it. Next, the athlete shifts the feet rapidly, moving each foot to the opposite side of the line. He continues the drill by changing the position of the feet with a scissorlike motion.

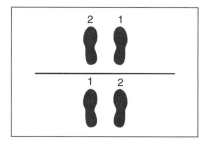

Forward and Backward Line Hops (Traveling Laterally)

LEVEL 1

The athlete stands with shoulders parallel to the line and then hops forward and backward over it with feet together. At the same time, he moves laterally down the line for a specified time period or predetermined distance. The athlete should travel to both the right and left sides to ensure balanced training.

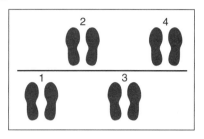

Lateral Line Hops (Traveling Forward and Backward)

LEVEL 1

The athlete stands with shoulders perpendicular to the line and then hops side to side over it with feet together. He moves forward down the line, hopping from side to side, until he reaches the end, and then returns to the starting position by hopping backward and side to side. This is done for a specified time period or a predetermined distance. The athlete should keep both feet together for the duration of the drill.

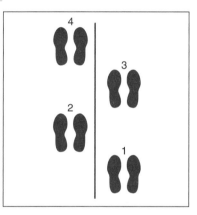

Single-Leg Variation

Hopping side to side over the line can also be performed on one leg. The athlete should complete the drill for a specified time period or number of repetitions. The drill should be performed equally on each leg to ensure balanced training.

Traveling Scissors

LEVEL 1

The athlete stands with shoulders parallel to the line and then steps across the line to straddle it with one foot in front of the line and the other behind it. He rapidly alternates the position of the feet, moving them forward and backward in a scissorlike motion while moving laterally down the line for a specified time period or a predetermined distance. This drill should be performed to both the right and left sides to ensure balanced training.

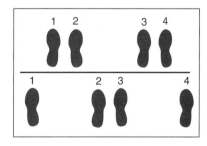

180-Degree Traveling Line Hop

LEVEL 2

The athlete stands on the line with shoulders and hips parallel to it. Next, he hops to the side while rotating the body 180 degrees in the air, landing on the line facing the opposite direction. He continues hopping and traveling laterally down the line for a specified time period or a predetermined distance. Both feet must land on the line for each hop.

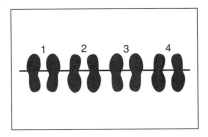

Single-Leg Variation

This drill can also be performed on one leg. As with the two-footed version, the athlete hops down the line, rotating the body 180 degrees with each hop. The foot must land on the line with each hop. This drill should be executed equally on each leg to ensure balanced training. The athlete performs the drill for a specified time period or a predetermined distance.

Using Alternative Patterns

Using alternative patterns can increase the complexity of these basic line drills and reduce the risk of boredom. The basic structure of each of the drills is unchanged, but instead of using a straight line, athletes can perform the drill around other shapes (see figure 4.1) to add challenge and variety. Possible options include a zigzag line, a rectangle, an oval, a triangle, or a double line.

Adding a line (figure 4.1e) can increase the intensity and metabolic demand of each drill. For example, in the forward and backward line hops, athletes can jump with both feet over the first line, then over the second line. Without pausing, they can immediately jump backward over the second line and then the first. Coaches should place the lines approximately 12 to 18 inches (30–46 cm) apart. If athletes cannot maintain balance, stability, and body position, the distance between the lines can be shortened. Coaches should increase the distance when athletes are able to manage a greater work load.

Adding Auditory or Visual Stimuli

Coaches can add external stimuli to any of these drills to create a reactionary component. For example, a partner or coach can call out random directional cues (e.g., *change directions* or *stop*) during the line drills, and the athlete must respond quickly and effectively. Moreover, coaches can introduce visual stimuli for greater sport specificity. An example is periodically tossing a ball to an athlete during a drill. To challenge cognitive decision making, coaches

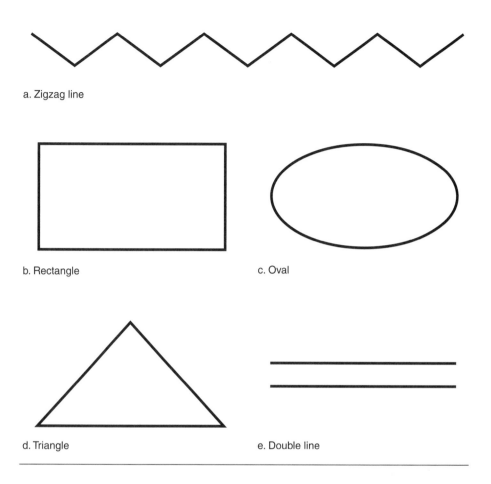

a. Zigzag line

b. Rectangle

c. Oval

d. Triangle

e. Double line

Figure 4.1 Alternative line patterns.

can prearrange several field markers and require the athlete to immediately stop what he is doing and sprint to a cone when prompted by a visual or verbal cue.

LADDER DRILLS

Coaches commonly use ladder drills to help athletes develop quick feet, body control, and kinesthetic awareness, as well as improve fundamental movement skills. Most agility ladders are made of plastic rungs that are attached to nylon straps to form boxes. Typically, the boxes are set approximately 12 to 18 inches (30–46 cm) apart. However, the box size can be adjusted by sliding the rungs up or down the nylon straps. Coaches may wish to periodically alter the size of each box so that athletes are forced to adjust their stride length and foot placement. Making these adjustments in foot placement mimics the action requirements of competition. Generally, an athlete makes one complete pass by going down the ladder, leading with one foot, and then coming back, leading with the other. This ensures equal training. Coaches can adjust passes to meet the needs of an athlete or the team. (See chapter 6 for recommendations on volume and intensity.)

When performing these drills, athletes must progress from drills that are simple to those that are more complex. Initially, they should focus on performing each drill as fast as they can, not as fast as they can't! In other words, athletes should perform each drill as quickly as possible without hindering proper body control or position.

One in the Hole

LEVEL 1

The athlete stands at the end of the ladder with shoulders and hips parallel to the rungs and then steps into the first box of the ladder with one foot. Next, he steps in the following box with the opposite foot and repeats the process down the ladder. The athlete repeats this drill, this time leading with the opposite foot.

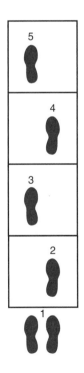

Two in the Hole

LEVEL 1

The athlete stands at the end of the ladder with the shoulders and hips parallel to the rungs. The athlete steps into the first box with one foot and then steps into the same box with the other foot. This pattern is continued through the ladder. The athlete should alternate the lead foot on subsequent trials.

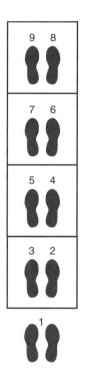

Lateral Two in the Hole

LEVEL 1

The athlete stands sideways at the end of the ladder so that the hips and shoulders are perpendicular to the rungs. With the foot closest to the ladder, he steps into the first box and then steps the other foot into the same box, placing it next to the lead foot. The athlete should not cross the legs. He continues by moving laterally down the ladder, stepping first with the lead foot and then moving the other foot into the same box. The athlete repeats this drill, leading with the opposite foot.

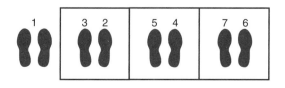

Skip

LEVEL 1

Skips can be used to increase the complexity of one in the hole, two in the hole, and lateral two in the hole. To perform this variation, the athlete steps into each box using a skip-step, or step-hop, pattern. A skip pattern requires the athlete to take off and land with the same leg. In contrast, regular patterns require athletes to alternate legs between takeoff and landing. Before doing a skip pattern in the speed ladder, coaches should make sure the athlete can skip 10 to 15 yards (10–15 m).

Cha-Cha

LEVEL 1

The athlete stands to the side of the first box with shoulders and hips perpendicular to the sides of the ladder. With the leg closest to the ladder, he steps laterally into the far half of first box and then steps the other foot into the same box. With the first leg, the athlete then steps to the outside of the ladder (opposite side of the starting point) and follows with the trailing foot. The athlete takes another step to the side with the first leg and then steps diagonally into the far half of the second box, leading with what was previously the trailing foot. Now, he steps into the second box with the trailing leg (formerly the leading leg). The athlete continues this pattern to the end of the ladder, stepping into and out of the boxes and switching the leading leg all the way through.

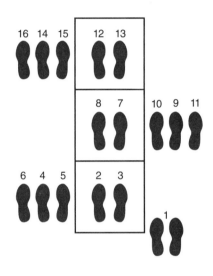

Ickey Shuffle

LEVEL 1

The athlete stands to the side of the first box with hips and shoulders perpendicular to the sides of the ladder. With the foot closest to the ladder, he steps laterally into the far half of the first box and then immediately steps the other foot into the box. Next, the athlete steps outside of the box on the other side with the lead foot and then steps with the other foot into the next box. This step is immediately followed by the outside foot. The athlete performs the same pattern of stepping out on the other side of the ladder. He continues this pattern down the ladder, alternating legs and sides of the ladder. To further challenge kinesthetic awareness and movement proficiency, the athlete can perform this drill moving backward.

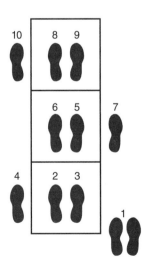

Carioca

LEVEL 1

The athlete stands at the end of the ladder with hips and shoulders perpendicular to the rungs. With the foot farthest from the ladder, he steps laterally into box 1 by crossing the outside foot in front of the other leg. The athlete steps into box 2 by moving the trailing leg behind and beyond the original lead leg. Next, he steps into box 3 with the original leading leg, crossing it behind the foot in box 2. The athlete steps into box 4 by moving the foot from box 2 in front of the other leg and to the side. He continues moving laterally, alternating the front and back movement of the trailing leg. The athlete then repeats the drill, leading with the opposite foot.

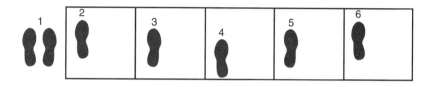

Billy Sims Crossover: In and Two Steps Out

LEVEL 1

The athlete stands to the side of box 1 with the hips and shoulders perpendicular to the sides of the ladder. He crosses the outer leg in front of the other to step into the center of box 1. The athlete then moves the other leg behind the lead leg, across the ladder, and outside the first box. This movement is followed quickly by the first leg. Next, the athlete crosses the outside leg over to step into the center of box 2. This pattern is repeated down the ladder. The athlete should take two steps to the outside of each box and should do a crossover step into the center of each one.

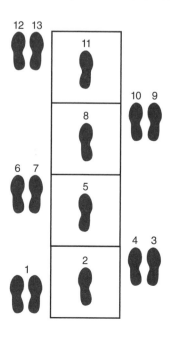

Hopscotch

LEVEL 1

The athlete stands with the feet straddling the first box of the ladder. The left foot is on the left side and the right foot is on the right side. The hips and shoulders should be parallel to the rungs. The athlete quickly hops into box 1, landing on one foot. After landing, he immediately hops forward, landing so that the feet straddle box 2. Then, the athlete quickly hops into box 2, landing on the other foot. The athlete continues this pattern down the ladder, hopping with both feet outside the ladder and alternating the landing foot inside the boxes.

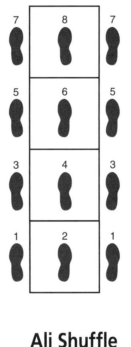

Ali Shuffle

LEVEL 1

The athlete stands to one side of box 1, which is formed by the first and second rungs of the ladder. The hips and shoulders should be perpendicular to the rungs. The athlete hops, moving the foot closest to the end of the ladder into box 1 and the other foot to the side. Using a scissorlike motion, he hops again, stepping the foot behind the ladder into box 2 and moving the original lead foot behind box 2. The athlete continues, switching feet and travelling laterally down the ladder. This drill should be completed in both directions (alternating the lead leg) to ensure balanced training.

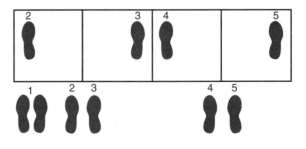

Lateral One in the Hole

LEVEL 1

The athlete stands to one side of box 1 between the first and second rungs of the ladder. The hips and shoulders should be perpendicular to the rungs. The athlete touches the foot closest to the second rung in and out of the center of box 1. Then he shuffles laterally to the outside of box 2, leading with the same foot. He again taps the lead foot in and out of box 2 and continues to shuffle laterally down the ladder, touching the lead foot into each box. The athlete repeats this drill facing the opposite direction, leading with the other foot and placing it in each box.

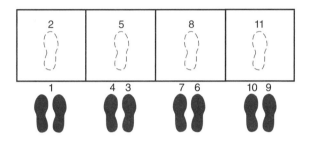

Two In, Two Out (Traveling Laterally)

LEVEL 1

The athlete stands to the side of the first box with the hips and shoulders perpendicular to the rungs. With the foot closest to the second rung, he steps into the center of box 1. The other foot follows immediately. As the second foot enters the box, the athlete steps the first foot back out diagonally to face box 2. The other foot follows immediately. The athlete shuffles down the ladder laterally, placing both feet in turn in each box of the ladder. The athlete repeats this drill in the opposite direction, switching lead legs.

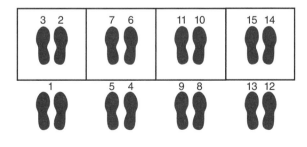

Slaloms

LEVEL 2

The athlete stands to the side of the first box with the hips and shoulders parallel to the rungs. He hops with both feet into the center of box 1 and then immediately hops with both feet out of the box to the other side. Next, the athlete hops diagonally with both feet into the center of box 2 and then immediately hops out diagonally with both feet on the other side, landing at the top of the box. This zigzag pattern is continued down the ladder. This drill may also be performed laterally or backward.

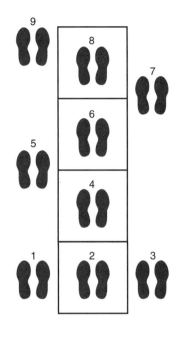

Cherry Pickers

LEVEL 2

The athlete stands at the end of the ladder with hips and shoulders parallel to the rungs. He hops forward and lands with one foot outside box 1 and the other foot in the center of it. The athlete bends forward, reaches down with the hand opposite the foot in the box, and touches the ground directly in front of the foot in the box. The athlete then hops into box 2, switching the leg position so that the outside leg goes to the center of the box and the inside leg lands outside it. He bends down and again touches the ground in front of the leg in the box with the opposite arm. The athlete continues this drill down the ladder, alternating foot and hand positions. This drill can also be performed moving backward.

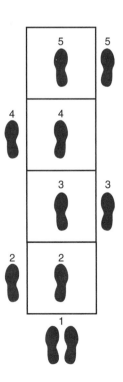

180s

The athlete stands with the feet straddling the first rung of the ladder. The hips and shoulders should be perpendicular to the rungs. The athlete jumps to the side, rotating 180 degrees, and lands straddling the next rung. This pattern is continued down the ladder.

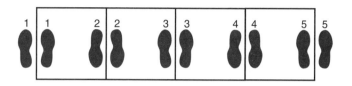

DOT DRILLS

Athletes commonly use dot drills to improve foot speed and kinesthetic awareness. To set up a basic pattern for dot drills, place five dots in an X. This can be done with tape or spray paint on the ground or on a workout surface in a training facility. Each dot should be approximately 4 inches (10 cm) in diameter. The dots that make up the perimeter should be placed 3 feet (1 m) apart, as shown in figure 4.2. The dots are numbered as follows: The center dot is 1, the top left corner as the athlete looks at the square is 2, the right top corner is 3, the bottom left corner is 4, and the bottom right corner is 5.

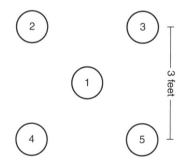

Figure 4.2 Basic dot drill pattern.

These drills involve three phases: (1) landing, (2) amortization (ground contact), and (3) takeoff. The landing phase starts as soon as the muscles begin to experience an eccentric movement. The rapid eccentric stretch of the muscle subsequently activates the stretching reflex. Thus, athletes should have good eccentric strength during the landing phase. Inadequate strength results in a slow rate of stretching and less activation of the stretching reflex.

The amortization phase is the time spent on the ground, or the amount of time between landing and takeoff. This phase is crucial for speed development. If the amortization phase is too long, the stretching reflex will dissipate as heat. Athletes will lose the benefit of using stored elastic energy to help forcefully propel the body. The takeoff phase includes the concentric action (shortening of the muscle fibers) that follows amortization. During this phase, athletes use stored elastic energy to increase jumping height, speed of movement, and distance traveled.

Dot drills are often called *multiple-response drills* because they involve repeated performance of either single- or double-leg movements. These drills often include a change of direction or body orientation. Various levels of intensity exist in the category of multiple-response drills:

▶ *Simple* multiple-response drills involve repeatedly moving forward and backward or side to side on both legs. Although these types of drills are relatively easy to perform, they set the stage for more difficult progressions. The primary focus of these drills is to develop sport-specific kinesthetic awareness and the ability to quickly change direction with control.

▶ *Intermediate* multiple-response drills incorporate forward, backward, and side-to-side movement patterns within the same drill. The objective of these drills is to perform them as quickly as possible while maintaining proper body position. As athletes advance with more complex drills, they should still focus on changing direction as quickly as possible with control.

▶ *Advanced* dot drills allow for the greatest neurological adaptations. Athletes perform these drills with a single leg. This may allow for the development of better speed (both unilaterally and overall) and agility.

The drills in this section involve combinations of double-leg jumping movements that can improve an athlete's ability to change directions and react. The athlete should start in a good athletic position with the feet close together. As he moves through the drill, he works to maintain this position with balance and control. To increase the skill level of simple drills (those that use only forward and backward or lateral movements) to intermediate, coaches may add the missing directional movement (forward and backward or lateral) to the drill pattern. To increase the level to advanced, athletes can perform the patterns on one leg.

Forward and Back
LEVEL 1

This basic foot-speed drill focuses on rapid forward and backward changes of direction. The pattern for this drill is 4-2-4 or 5-3-5, starting from the first dot in each pattern.

Diagonal Jumps
LEVEL 1

The purpose of this drill is to develop rapid change-of-direction speed while moving forward, backward, and diagonally. The patterns for this drill are 2-1-5-1-2 and 3-1-4-1-3. Athletes should perform both patterns to ensure balanced training.

V Drill
LEVEL 1

This is a basic foot-speed drill that focuses on forward, backward, and diagonal changes of direction. The pattern for this drill is 1-2-1-3, starting at dot 1.

Arrow Drill
LEVEL 1

This is a basic foot-speed drill that focuses on forward, backward, and diagonal changes of direction. The pattern for this drill is 1-4-1-5, starting at dot 1.

M Drill
LEVEL 1

The purpose of this drill is to develop foot speed in forward, backward, lateral, and diagonal patterns. The pattern for this drill is 4-2-1-3-5. The athlete repeats this drill in reverse, using a 5-3-1-2-4 pattern to change the direction of movement. The athlete starts on the dot listed first in the pattern and faces the same direction throughout the duration of each drill pattern.

Figure Eight

LEVEL 1

The purpose of this drill is to improve kinesthetic awareness and change-of-direction speed. The pattern for this drill is 2-3-1-4-5-1-2. The athlete repeats this drill in reverse, using a 2-1-5-4-1-3-2 pattern to change the direction of the movement. The athlete starts at dot 2 each time.

Hopscotch

LEVEL 1

The athlete starts with one foot on dot 4 and the other on dot 5, facing dots 1, 2, and 3. He jumps and lands with both feet on dot 1. The athlete jumps forward again and lands with split feet on dots 2 and 3. The athlete repeats this pattern, hopping backward to return to the starting position.

CONE DRILLS

Coaches typically use cones as landmarks to set up a variety of preprogrammed agility drills. The purpose of each drill in this section is to improve movement through a series of preplanned directional changes. Coaches can also revise them into semiopen drills by creating movement options and having the athlete respond to an external stimulus.

Two-Cone Drills

Coaches place two cones apart from one another at a set distance that works best for their sport or activity. In most situations, a distance of 5 to 10 yards (5–9 m) is adequate. Athletes can perform numerous drills with this setup to improve basic changes of directions. The following are just a few suggestions.

Forward Run

LEVEL 1

The athlete starts in front of cone 1. When ready, he sprints forward to cone 2. When the athlete reaches it, he comes to a complete stop in the athletic position, then immediately turns and accelerates in the opposite direction. The athlete sprints past cone 1.

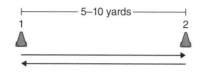

Backpedal

LEVEL 1

The athlete starts just in front of cone 1, facing away from the cones. When ready, he backpedals to cone 2. When the athlete reaches it, he immediately turns and backpedals to cone 1. The focus of this drill should be on keeping the hips low and maintaining the athletic position.

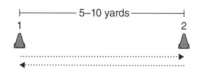

Lateral Shuffle

LEVEL 1

The athlete starts in an athletic position facing cone 1. When ready, he shuffles to cone 2, keeping the hips low and the hips, shoulders, and torso parallel to the cones. When he reaches cone 2, the athlete immediately shuffles back to cone 1. The feet should not cross during this drill.

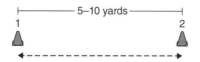

Carioca

LEVEL 1

The athlete starts in an athletic position facing cone 1. Keeping the hips low, she moves laterally by crossing the trail leg in front of the other leg (photo *a*), stepping out with the lead leg (photo *b*), crossing behind with the trail leg (photo *c*), stepping out with the lead leg, and so on. The athlete should keep the hips, shoulders, and torso parallel to the cones. When the athlete reaches cone 2, she should repeat the movement back to cone 1, using the opposite leg for the crossover and cross-behind steps.

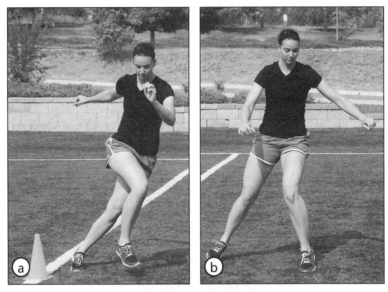

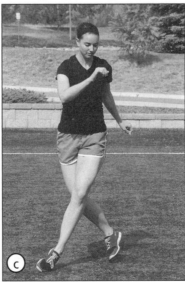

Power Carioca

LEVEL 1

The athlete performs this drill in the same manner as the carioca except that he forcefully drives the knee upward when the leg crosses in front of the body (photo *a*). The thigh should be parallel with the ground at the highest position. As with the regular carioca, the athlete steps out with the lead leg (right leg in this case; photo *b*) and crosses the trail leg behind (photo *c*).

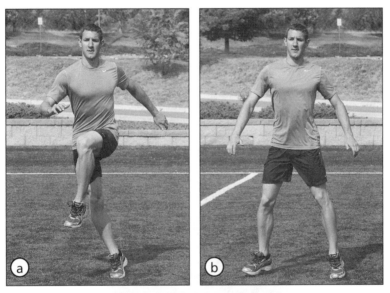

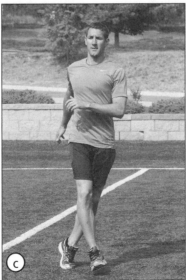

180-Degree Drill

LEVEL 2

The athlete starts beside cone 1 and then sprints to cone 2. When he reaches it, he uses short, choppy steps to round the cone and then accelerates back to cone 1. When rounding the cone, the athlete should stay as close to it as possible. This is done by shifting the body's center of mass toward the turning side. The athlete should repeat the drill, performing turns to both the right and the left.

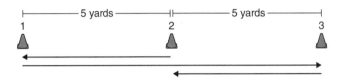

Once the athlete has mastered the technique in these basic drills, the coach can combine each of these tasks in different ways to create a wide variety of movement patterns, such as progressing from simple discrete movements (one movement) to serial tasks (a combination of movements). The examples of movement combinations that follow are level 2 drills. The athlete can add more variety by touching each cone with the preferred hand.

▶ The athlete sprints forward to cone 2 and then backpedals to cone 1.

▶ The athlete sprints forward to cone 2 and then shuffles back to cone 1.

▶ The athlete shuffles to cone 2 and then backpedals to cone 1.

▶ The athlete shuffles to cone 2 and then sprints back to cone 1.

▶ The athlete shuffles first to cone 2 and then back to cone 1. He turns 90 degrees and sprints past cone 2.

▶ The athlete backpedals to cone 2 and then sprints back to cone 1.

▶ The athlete backpedals to cone 2 and then shuffles back to cone 1.

▶ The athlete performs the carioca or power carioca to cone 2 and then turns and sprints back to cone 1.

Three-Cone Drills

Adding a third cone allows for different combinations of movements and increases the complexity of the drills. To set up for three-cone drills, coaches should place three cones in a straight line, spaced approximately 5 yards (5 m) apart.

While performing three-cone drills, athletes must maintain a good athletic position. They should also use short, choppy steps to round the cones. The 180-degree drill in the previous section provides good training for three-cone drills. Athletes can use a variety of movement combinations for three-cone drills. Additionally, all of the drills in the previous section can be modified for three cones. The following examples are just some of the possible combinations for three-cone drills. All are level 2 drills.

- ▶ The athlete sprints forward to cone 2, turns 180 degrees, and backpedals to cone 3.
- ▶ The athlete sprints forward to cone 2, turns 90 degrees, and shuffles to cone 3. He repeats this drill, facing the opposite direction during the shuffle.
- ▶ The athlete sprints forward to cone 2, performs a 360-degree turn around it, and sprints to cone 3.
- ▶ The athlete shuffles to cone 2, turns 90 degrees, and backpedals to cone 3.
- ▶ The athlete shuffles to cone 2 and then back to cone 1, then immediately turns 90 degrees and sprints past cone 3.
- ▶ The athlete backpedals to cone 2, turns 180 degrees, and then sprints past cone 3.
- ▶ The athlete backpedals to cone 2, turns 90 degrees, and then shuffles past cone 3. He repeats this drill, facing the opposite direction during the shuffle.

Coaches can also use drills created specifically for three cones. Some drills presented here use the basic cone setup discussed previously and others use different layouts.

Pro-Agility Drill
LEVEL 2

This drill is often used to test change-of-direction speed and agility. It also improves agility performance. Coaches should use the basic three-cone setup. The athlete begins facing cone 2, with the hips, shoulders, and torso parallel to the cones. When ready, or on the *go* signal, the athlete turns and sprints left to cone 1, turns 180 degrees and sprints back to cone 3, makes another 180-degree turn, then sprints back past the middle cone. This drill can be performed in either direction.

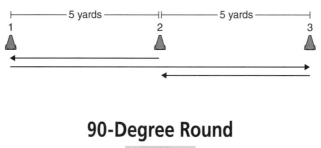

90-Degree Round
LEVEL 1

This beginning movement pattern teaches body position, body control, and how to adjust to forces during movement. Three cones are set up in an *L* shape, with legs 10 yards (9 m) long. The athlete starts inside of cone 1, keeping the hips, shoulders, and torso parallel to the cone. When ready, he turns and sprints toward cone 2. As he approaches it, the athlete slows down slightly, moves to the outside, and makes a 90-degree turn around cone 2. He then accelerates out of the turn and then sprints past cone 3.

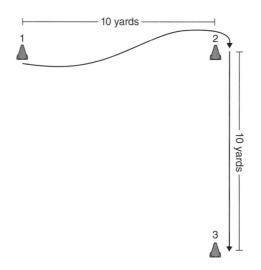

90-Degree Cut

LEVEL 2

The purpose of this drill is to develop quick transitions between high-speed agility movements. Three cones are set up in an *L* shape, with legs 10 yards (9 m) long (figure *a*). The athlete starts outside of cone 1, keeping the hips, shoulders, and torso in line with the cone. When ready, he sprints to cone 2. As he reaches it, the athlete drops down into a good athletic position, makes a sharp lateral cut (*b* and *c*), and sprints past cone 3. This drill should be performed in both directions for an equal number of repetitions.

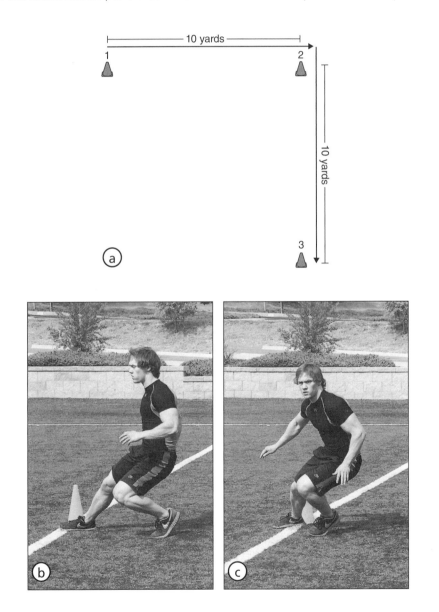

L Drill

LEVEL 2

The purpose of this drill is to maintain sport-specific balance and the ability to accelerate during quick directional changes. Three cones are set up in an *L* shape, with legs 10 yards (9 m) long. The athlete starts outside of cone 1. He sprints from cone 1 to cone 2 and then drops down into an athletic position by slowing down, lowering the center of gravity, and squaring up the feet. The athlete then performs a sharp 90-degree cut and accelerates to cone 3. He makes a 180-degree turn around cone 3 using short, choppy steps and then accelerates back to cone 2. The athlete makes another sharp 90-degree cut and sprints back to cone 1. Coaches can set up this drill to be run in the opposite direction.

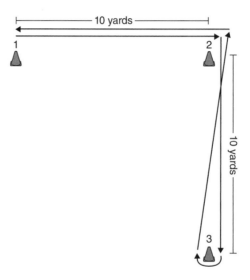

T Drill

LEVEL 2

Three cones are set up in a straight line, with each cone 5 yards (5 m) apart from the next. These are cones 2, 3 and 4. A fourth cone (cone 1) is placed perpendicular to cone 3, about 10 yards (9 m) away. (Although this drill technically uses four cones, it fits with the three-cone drills because the first cone is used only as a starting point.) The resulting *T* pattern is commonly used to develop rapid acceleration, deceleration, and explosive change of direction. Starting at cone 1, the athlete sprints to cone 3, cuts left, and then sprints to cone 2. Using short, choppy steps, the athlete performs a 180-degree turn around cone 2, and then sprints to cone 4. He then performs a 180-degree turn around cone 4 and sprints back to cone 3. He cuts left and then accelerates past the starting cone.

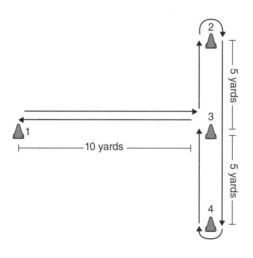

Four-Cone Drills

As athletes advance in their progressions, they should add a variety of movement patterns, including forward, backward, and lateral movements, as well as different angles, such as a 45-degree lateral drop. Adding landmarks (cones) increases the complexity of the drills and requires more mobility and body control, since athletes move in multiple directions and accelerate and decelerate in different patterns. The following drills require four cones set up in a square. Each side of the square should be 10 to 15 yards (9–14 m) long.

Square Run

LEVEL 2

The athlete starts in an athletic position outside of cone 1, with the hips, shoulders, and torso perpendicular to the cone. When ready, or on a cue, he sprints to cone 2. When the athlete reaches it, he breaks down into athletic position, makes a 90-degree cut, and then sprints to cone 3. He continues this pattern around all the cones until he reaches cone 1 again. This drill should be run in both the clockwise and counterclockwise directions. The athlete can also run backward or shuffle laterally through the cones.

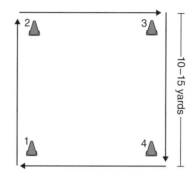

Four Corners Drill

LEVEL 2

The athlete starts in an athletic position outside of cone 1, with the hips, shoulders, and torso perpendicular to it. When ready, or on a cue, he sprints to cone 2 and then shuffles to cone 3. Next, the athlete backpedals to cone 4. Finally, he shuffles back to cone 1 to finish the drill.

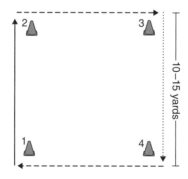

Lateral Bear Crawl and Backpedal Drill

LEVEL 2

This drill uses a pattern similar to that of the four corners drill, but a lateral bear crawl replaces the shuffle. The athlete starts in an athletic position outside of cone 1, with the hips, shoulders, and torso perpendicular to it. When ready, or on a cue, he sprints to cone 2. While continuing to face the same direction, the athlete assumes a bear-crawl position (see photo *b*) and moves laterally to cone 3. At cone 3, he stands as quickly as possible and backpedals to cone 4. Here, the athlete returns to the ground and bear crawls laterally back to cone 1, continuing to face the same direction.

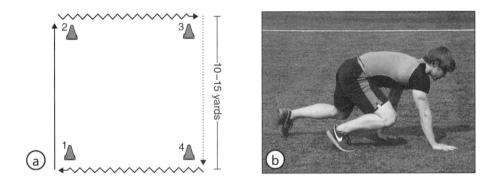

Tic-Tac-Toe Drill

LEVEL 2

The athlete starts in an athletic position with the hips, shoulders, and torso perpendicular to cone 1. When ready, or on a cue, he sprints to cone 2. Here, he breaks down into an athletic position, cuts laterally, and sprints to cone 3. Next, the athlete circles cone 3 and then sprints to cone 4. He circles cone 4 and then shuffles to cone 1. The athlete should repeat this drill in the opposite direction to ensure balanced training, starting at cone 4.

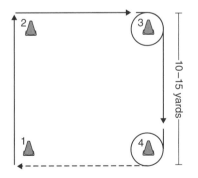

360-Degree Drill

LEVEL 2

The athlete starts in an athletic position on the outside of cone 1, with the hips, shoulders, and torso perpendicular to it. When ready, or on a cue, he sprints to cone 2. When he reaches it, the athlete slows down slightly and makes a 360-degree turn around cone 2. He repeats this same pattern around cones 3 and 4, and then sprints back to cone 1. The athlete should also move around the cones in the opposite direction to ensure balanced training.

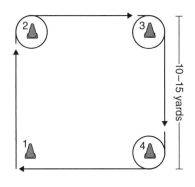

X Drill

LEVEL 2

The athlete starts in an athletic position outside of cone 1, with the hips, shoulders, and torso perpendicular to it. When ready, or on a cue, he sprints to cone 2. The athlete backpedals around it and continues to backpedal diagonally to cone 4. At cone 4, the athlete plants, turns, and sprints around it, and then runs forward to cone 3. At cone 3, the athlete backpedals around it and continues to backpedal diagonally to cone 1 to finish the drill. The movement pattern in this drill can be varied by starting with a sprint and then performing a shuffle.

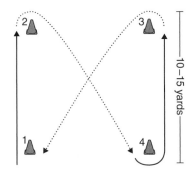

Five-Cone Drills

Five-cone drills once again add more landmarks, increasing the complexity of movement, the demands on body position, proper agility form, and technique. The drills in this section require four cones set up in a square with one cone in the center. The cones around the perimeter are numbered 1 through 4, and cone 5 is in the middle. The sides of the square should be 10 to 15 yards (9–14 m) long.

M Drill

LEVEL 2

The athlete starts in an athletic position outside of cone 1, with the hips, shoulders, and torso perpendicular to it. When ready, or on a cue, he sprints to cone 2. After reaching it, the athlete breaks down into an athletic position and plants the outside foot to change direction as he passes the cone. From cone 2, the athlete shuffles diagonally to cone 5, then breaks down into an athletic position, plants one foot, and then sprints to cone 3. After reaching it, the athlete breaks down into an athletic position, plants the outside foot, and then backpedals to cone 4. After passing it, the athlete plants, and then shuffles laterally back to cone 1. This drill should be performed in both directions to ensure balanced training.

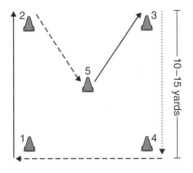

Star Drill

LEVEL 2

The athlete stands outside of cone 1, facing the center of the box. He should continue to face this direction throughout the drill. On the *start* command, he sprints diagonally to cone 5, backpedals back to cone 1, and then shuffles to cone 2. At cone 2, the athlete turns and sprints diagonally to cone 5, backpedals to cone 2, and then shuffles to cone 3. Next, he sprints diagonally to cone 5, backpedals to cone 3, and then shuffles to cone 4. At cone 4, the athlete turns, sprints diagonally to cone 5, and then backpedals to cone 4. To finish the drill, he shuffles from cone 4 to cone 1. The athlete should perform this drill in the opposite direction and change the movement pattern. For example, he could start by shuffling to cone 5 and then sprint backward to each cone in the pattern.

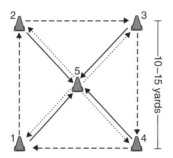

Star Drill With Bear Crawl

LEVEL 2

This variation of the star drill develops total-body agility. The athlete stands in an athletic position at cone 1 facing the center of the box. On the *start* command, he sprints diagonally to cone 5 and then bear crawls back to cone 1. The athlete then stands and shuffles to cone 2 while facing the center of the box. At cone 2, he turns and sprints diagonally to cone 5 and then bear crawls back to cone 2. Next, he stands and shuffles to cone 3 while facing the center. The athlete sprints diagonally to cone 5, assumes a bear-crawl position as quickly as possible, and moves back to cone 3. He returns to a standing position and shuffles to cone 4, facing the center of the box. The athlete turns and sprints diagonally to cone 5 and then bear crawls back to cone 4. To finish the drill, he stands again and shuffles to cone 1. The athlete should reverse the direction to change shuffle and movement patterns.

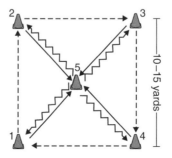

Butterfly Drill

LEVEL 2

The athlete stands in an athletic position at cone 1, facing the center of the box. On the *start* command, he sprints diagonally to cone 5. Next, he shuffles to cone 2, leading with the left leg. The athlete sprints around it and then continues sprinting to cone 5. Next, he shuffles to cone 3, again leading with the left leg. The athlete sprints around cone 3 and continues to cone 5. He shuffles with the left lead leg to cone 4 and sprints around it and back to cone 5. To finish the drill, the athlete shuffles back to cone 1 (start), leading with the left leg. The athlete should repeat this drill, leading with the other leg on the shuffles.

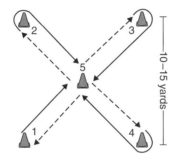

Hourglass Drill

LEVEL 2

The athlete starts in an athletic position at cone 1, facing the center of the box (figure *a*). On the *start* command, he performs carioca, leading with the right leg to cone 4. At cone 4, the athlete sprints diagonally to cone 5 and then turns and backpedals diagonally to cone 3. Next, he shuffles to cone 2, leading with the right leg and facing the center of the box and then sprints to cone 5. At cone 5, the athlete shuffles, leading with the left leg, to cone 3 (figure *b*), and then sprints back to cone 5. He then shuffles, leading with the left leg, to cone 4 and sprints back to cone 5. To finish the drill, the athlete shuffles, leading with the left leg, to cone 1. To alter the pattern, the athlete may change the lead leg on the shuffles and replace the sprinting to cone 5 with backpedaling.

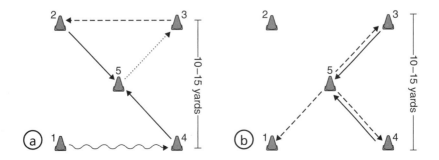

Attack and Retreat Drill

LEVEL 2

For this five-cone drill, the 5-yard (5 m) midway point between each pair of outside cones needs to be marked. The athlete starts in an athletic position outside cone 1. On the *start* command, the athlete faces outside the box and shuffles 5 yards toward cone 2. At the 5-yard mark, he plants and sprints to cone 5 and then returns to the same 5-yard mark by backpedaling. At the 5-yard mark, the athlete continues facing inside the box and shuffles to cone 2. At cone 2, he faces outside the box and shuffles to the 5-yard mark between cones 2 and 3. At the 5-yard mark, the athlete plants, sprints to cone 5, and then backpedals back to the 5-yard mark. The athlete faces inside the box and shuffles to cone 3. At cone 3, he turns to face outside the box, shuffles to the 5-yard mark between cones 3 and 4, plants at the 5-yard mark, sprints to cone 5, backpedals back to the 5-yard mark, and then faces inside the box and shuffles to cone 4. At cone 4, the athlete faces outside the box and shuffles to the 5-yard mark between cones 1 and 4, plants, sprints to cone 5, and backpedals back to the 5-yard mark. To finish the drill, the athlete faces inside the box and shuffles past cone 1.

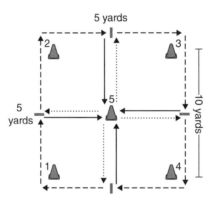

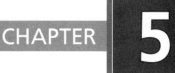

CHAPTER 5

Quickness Drills

Jay Dawes

Chapter 4 presents a variety of drills to improve speed and agility when changing direction. As previously stated, these drills are an excellent way to develop proper technique and form. However, since most sports are open in nature and occur in an ever-changing and often chaotic environment, sport-specific drills that require both perceptual and decision-making skills may better prepare athletes for competition. These quickness and reactive-type drills require athletes to accurately anticipate, read, and respond to various environmental stimuli to perform accurately and efficiently, as they would in an actual sporting event.

AGILITY-DRILL ADAPTATION

The variety of closed agility drills in chapter 4 focus on improving change-of-direction speed. After athletes become proficient at these drills, they can add several stimuli to change the drills' complexity, increasing the reactive demands. Thus, with a few small adaptations, virtually any agility drill can be made into a quickness drill. The following are examples of ways to progress many of the agility drills into reactive (quickness) drills using auditory and visual cues.

▶ *Auditory cues.* The coach may periodically give an auditory cue, such as *switch, change,* or *stop,* while the athlete is performing the drill. At this cue, the athlete should immediately and accurately respond. For instance, while an athlete is running forward, the coach gives the *back* command. The athlete responds by immediately decelerating and running back toward the starting line. Additional auditory cues and distracters may be added to agility drills to help the athlete focus in on task-relevant auditory information. For example, a football coach might use a snap count to signal the beginning of a drill. Keep in mind that reaction time is typically delayed when more auditory cues are added because the athletes must decipher among and respond to multiple stimuli. For this reason, coaches should limit possible response cues and distracters to two or three options.

▶ *Visual cues.* Coaches can use a variety of visual stimuli to increase the reactionary demands and sport specificity of virtually any agility drill. During competition, athletes must constantly scan the field for teammates, opponents, a ball or puck, a referee, or coach signals from the sidelines. For this reason, incorporating different types of visual stimuli and cues may help players more quickly identify task-relevant game cues during competition. These cues may be as simple as a coach or teammate pointing to a marker to prompt an immediate change in direction or a signal for the athlete to sprint forward and catch a dropped ball. They may also be as complex as reading an opponent's movements and responding accordingly.

▶ *Mixed cues.* Both auditory and visual cues may be combined to challenge even the most advanced athletes. For example, a football athlete randomly tosses a ball to the right or left side of someone running forward. As soon as the runner catches the ball, the coach calls out a number between 1 and 3. Each number corresponds to a cone. After catching the ball, the athlete runs to the specified cone to complete the drill. Initially, the runner must visually track the trajectory of the ball in order to receive it. Next, the athlete must listen for the coach's auditory cue to know where to run to complete the drill or play.

REACTION DRILLS

This section provides examples of quickness drills that improve the ability to identify a specific stimulus and to respond appropriately. Athletes must integrate a variety of auditory, visual, and sensory cues in order to execute each drill effectively. Once athletes consistently demonstrate good body control and technique, they can use these drills in a comprehensive agility-training program to improve reaction. This sort of program helps athletes quickly perform sport-specific tasks during competition.

Reactive Gear Drill

LEVEL 3

This drill develops first-step quickness and improves the ability to accelerate and decelerate. The athlete starts at one of two cones placed 20 yards (18 m) apart. On the coach's *go* signal, the athlete begins jogging back and forth between the two cones. (This speed is first gear.) When the coach calls *second gear,* the athlete speeds up to approximately three-fourths of full speed. When *third gear* is called, the athlete runs between the cones at full speed. The athlete should continue running between the cones for the entire duration of the drill (25 to 30 seconds).

To ensure that the athlete does not anticipate a specific gear, the coach should call out signals randomly. They should mix it up instead of repeatedly progressing through gears 1, 2, and 3 in order. For example, they might go from gear 1 to 3, followed by 2, or from 2 to 1 to 3. This keeps the drill unpredictable, forcing the athlete to focus intently on the auditory cues.

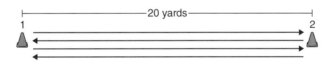

Reactive Sprint and Backpedal Drill

LEVEL 3

This drill improves the ability to accelerate and decelerate while running forward and backward, such as when covering an opponent in a variety of sports. Begin this drill by placing two cones 10 yards (9 m) apart. The athlete begins by standing in an athletic position at cone 1. On the *go* signal, the athlete runs forward toward cone 2. When the coach says *switch,* the athlete immediately decelerates and changes directions, backpedaling to cone 1.

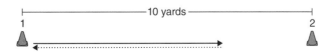

Wave Drill

LEVEL 3

Identifying visual signals from a teammate or coach during competition is an important skill. This drill enhances reactive quickness with visual cues. Two cones are placed 10 yards (9 m) apart. The athlete should stand in an athletic position at cone 1, and the coach should stand just behind cone 2. On the *go* command, the athlete begins chopping the feet and watching for the coach to give a visual signal for a directional change. To signal the athlete to run forward, the coach raises both arms overhead. The signal to run forward is always first. Once the athlete has reached the middle of the cones, the coach can change up the signals. To signal the athlete to backpedal, the coach drops both arms to the sides. The coach may also extend the arms directly in front to signal the athlete to stop in the current position, chop the feet, and wait for the next cue. The drill should last 8 to 10 seconds.

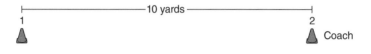

Shuffle Reaction Ball Drill

LEVEL 3

This drill improves lateral movement transitions and hand-eye coordination. Two cones are set up about 5 yards (5 m) apart. The athlete stands between the cones. The coach stands in front of the athlete and throws a ball toward either cone. The athlete must shuffle to the side to catch the ball and then toss it back. As the athlete's reaction time and movement patterns improve, the coach may increase the distance between the cones or the speed of the throw.

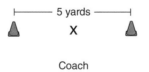

Ball Drops Drill

LEVEL 3

This drill is excellent for improving response to visual stimulus and first-step quickness. The athlete and coach stand approximately 5 yards (5 m) away from each other. The coach has a racquetball (or any ball that bounces). The athlete assumes an athletic position. The coach holds the ball out to the side at shoulder height and then randomly drops it. As soon as the coach releases the ball, the athlete sprints toward it and catches it before it bounces twice (see photo). The athlete should catch the ball in a good athletic stance. The athlete may not dive for the ball to make up for poor reaction time.

Variations

The coach and athlete can use the following variations to make the drill more challenging:

- Increase the distance between the athlete and the coach.
- Have the athlete start from different stances (three-point stance, on a knee, on the belly, and so on).
- The coach holds a ball on each side and drops only one. This requires the athlete to be aware of multiple focal points.
- The coach holds two balls and assigns a number to each (or uses different colored balls). Then, the coach drops both simultaneously while calling out a number (or color) to indicate which ball the athlete should attempt to catch.

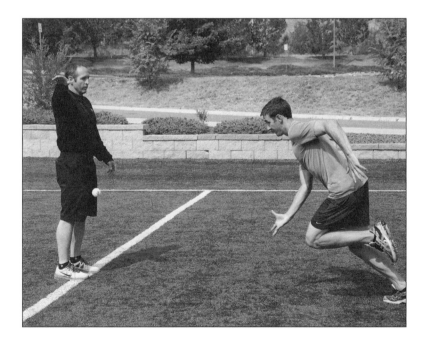

Shuffle and Forward Reaction Ball Drill

LEVEL 3

This is similar to the shuffle reaction ball drill, but it requires the athlete to move forward when reacting as well as side to side. One cone is placed in each corner of a square with sides about 5 yards (5 m) long. The athlete stands between two cones on one side of the square. The coach stands facing the athlete on the opposite side of the square, just outside the boundary. The coach throws a ball toward any of the four cones. The athlete reacts by shuffling to the side or moving forward to catch the ball, and then tosses it back to the coach. As the athlete's reaction time and movement patterns improve, the coach may increase the distance between the cones or the frequency of the throw.

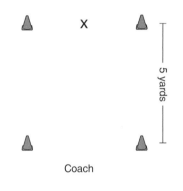

Triangle Drill

LEVEL 3

This drill improves fundamental quickness skills and reaction time by using an auditory stimulus. Three cones, numbered 1 through 3, are placed in a triangular pattern. The athlete stands in an athletic position at cone 1. The coach stands to the side and calls out a number that corresponds to one of the two cones in front of the athlete (see photo). The athlete immediately sprints to the chosen cone. Variations of this drill include the player facing away from the cones (forcing her to turn and open the hips) or beginning in a push-up position with hands flat on the floor and arms extended. This forces her to quickly scramble to her feet and explode forward toward the selected cone.

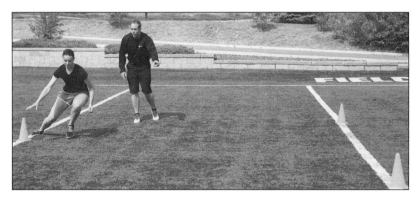

The athlete responds to auditory stimulus.

Jump, Squat, Push-Up Drill

LEVEL 3

This drill develops total-body quickness and reaction time. The athlete begins in an athletic position. The coach calls out *jump, squat,* or *push-up,* and the athlete must perform the exercise indicated. The athlete performs this drill for a total time of 10 seconds per set, resting for 20 to 50 seconds between sets.

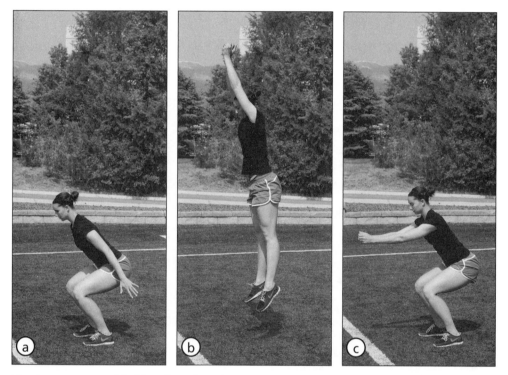

The jump starts with (*a*) a deep bend and ends with (*b*) a full extension of the body. (*c*) For the squat, the athlete sits back, leading with the hips and keeping the whole of each foot in contact with the ground.

Quickness Box

LEVEL 3

This drill is good for improving quickness in confined spaces. Four cones are set up to create a square with sides approximately 6 to 10 feet (2–3 m) long. The cones are numbered 1 through 4. The athlete assumes an athletic position in the center of the box (photo *a*) and waits for the coach to call out the number of one of the cones. When the coach signals, the athlete runs, backpedals (photo *b*), or shuffles as needed to touch the cone with either the closest hand or the one specified prior to starting the drill. After touching the cone, the athlete sprints back to the starting position and waits for the coach to call the next number. He repeats this drill for approximately 10 seconds per set and does two or three sets.

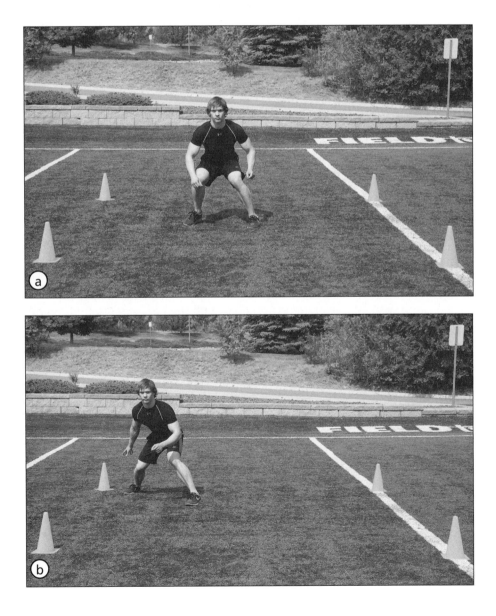

Y Drill

LEVEL 3

This drill teaches athletes to quickly adjust their stride and foot placement in order to transition into other movement patterns. Four cones are set up in a Y pattern (see illustration *a*). The two cones forming the top of the Y and the base cone should be placed about 10 yards (9 m) from the middle cone. The base cone is 1, the middle cone is 2, and the top cones are 3 and 4. The coach stands in front of cone 2 in the V at the top of the Y. The athlete assumes a sport-specific position at cone 1. On the coach's signal, the athlete sprints to cone 2. When the athlete reaches it, the coach gives a directional cue (see photo *b*) to signal which of the three cones the athlete should sprint to next. The directional cue can be a visual cue, such as pointing, or auditory cue, such as calling a number. The coach may modify this drill by having the athlete backpedal or side shuffle to the designated cone.

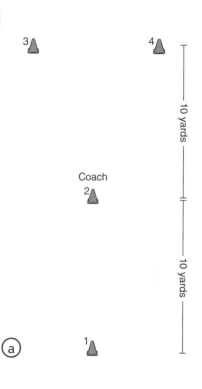

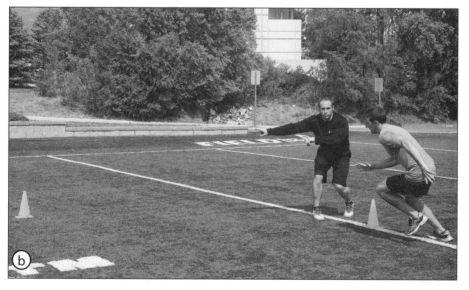

Number Drill

LEVEL 3

Six cones are positioned in two lines, approximately 10 yards (9 m) apart. Each cone in the line should be approximately 10 yards (9 m) away from the next. The first cones in both lines are 1, the middle cones are 2, and the last cones are 3. The athlete stands behind cone 1 in one of the lines. When the coach calls out a number, the athlete sprints to the corresponding cone in the opposite row of cones and stands by it, chopping the feet in place until the coach calls out the next directional cue. For each number the coach calls out, the athlete runs to the corresponding cone in the opposite line. The athlete continues this drill for 8 to 12 seconds, changing directions two to four times before resting. At least one set should be performed backward.

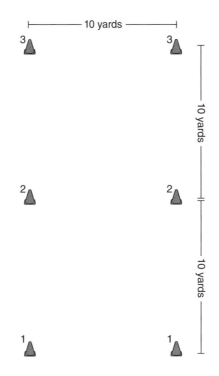

Reaction Race

LEVEL 3

This drill can improve motivation and add a competitive element to traditional quickness exercises. Six cones are positioned in two lines, approximately 3 to 5 yards (3–5 m) apart. The three cones in each line should be about 10 yards (9 m) away from one another. The coach should number the cones in each line 1 through 3 and draw a starting line in front of the number 1 cones. Two athletes choose their own line, then assume athletic positions approximately 5 yards behind the starting line and 3 feet (1 m) to the outside of their chosen row of cones. The coach starts the race by calling out a number. The athletes race to the corresponding cone in the line nearest them, touch the cone with one hand, turn, and sprint back through the starting line.

Variation

The coach may enhance the difficulty by using three sets of differently colored cones and randomly calling out either a number or a color for the athletes to respond to.

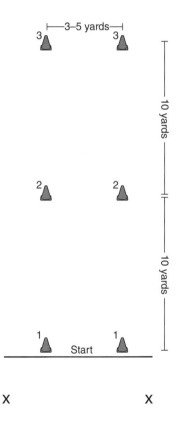

Get Up and Go

LEVEL 3

Six cones are positioned in two lines, approximately 10 to 15 yards (9–14 m) apart. The three cones in each line should be placed about 10 yards away from one another. The first cones in both lines are 1, the middle cones are 2, and the last cones are 3. This drill is very similar to the number drill. However, here, the athlete starts by lying on the belly behind and between the number 1 cones (photo a). When the coach calls out a number, the athlete sprints to the corresponding cone and drops down into a push-up position (or plank position with arms extended) at the new cone (photo c). As the drill continues, the athlete runs to the cone in the opposite line as designated by the coach's cue. The athlete continues this drill for 8 to 12 seconds, changing directions two to four times before resting. The set is repeated once.

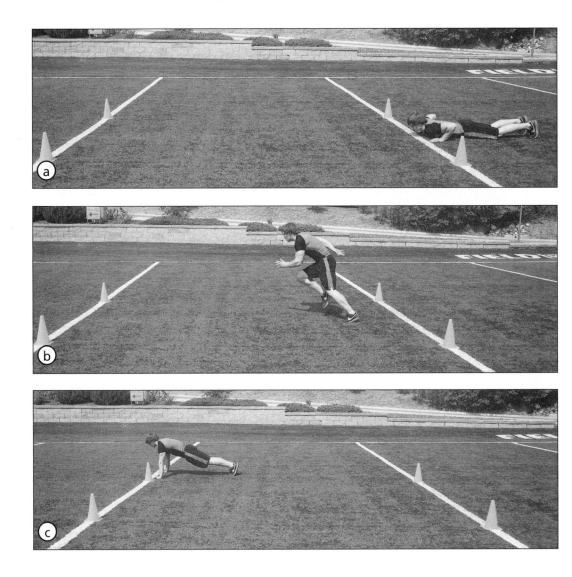

Shadow Drill

LEVEL 3

This drill teaches athletes to read an opponent's movement patterns. Two cones are set up 10 yards (9 m) apart from one another. Two athletes stand facing each other in the center of the cones. One athlete assumes the role of the leader. The other athlete must shadow the leader by mimicking his actions. For example, if the leader turns and sprints to a cone in his line, the other athlete sprints to the corresponding cone in the other line.

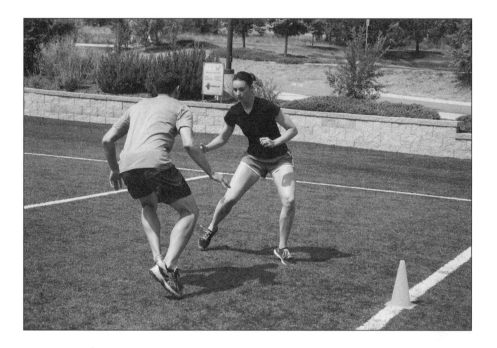

Coverage Drill

LEVEL 3

This drill teaches athletes to read the movement patterns of multiple opponents at the same time. Four cones are set up in a square, with sides 10 yards (9 m) long. One athlete starts in the center of the square. A second athlete lines up between a pair of cones and faces the athlete in the center. A third athlete lines up between the pair of cones to the left or right of the second athlete. On the *go* signal, the athletes along the perimeter of the square begin shuffling between the two cones on their sides of the square. The player in the center attempts to stay in alignment with (or squared up to) both athletes as they move between the cones. As the perimeter players move, the athlete in the center must adjust his position within the square as needed so he can keep both perimeter players in his field of vision. The athletes should perform this drill for approximately 10 seconds. After a 20- to 30-second rest, the athletes rotate to the left or right so that one of the perimeter athletes moves to the center. The drill must continue until each athlete has been in all three positions.

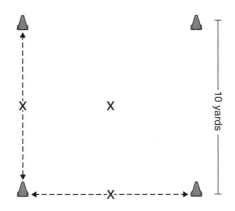

Gap Drill

This drill helps athletes find an opening to evade their competitors, such as in rugby or football. Four cones are set up approximately 1 yard (1 m) apart in a straight line to create three gaps, numbered 1 to 3. An athlete moves approximately 10 yards (9 m) away and assumes an athletic position facing the cones. On the *go* signal, the athlete runs forward. At the 5 to 8 yard (5–7 m) mark, the coach calls a gap number, and the athlete runs through the designated gap.

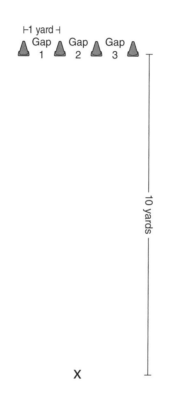

Containment Drill

LEVEL 3

This drill helps athletes improve sport-specific quickness and the ability to read and react to an opponent's movement patterns. Four cones are placed in a large square, with sides approximately 15 to 20 yards (14–18 m) long (see illustration a). The defensive player lines up between two cones on one side of the square, which becomes the end zone. The offensive player lines up between the cones on the opposite side of the square. On the *go* signal, the offensive player attempts to evade the defensive player (see photo *b*) and get into the end zone as quickly as possible. Although some physical contact will occur during this drill, athletes should not be overly aggressive or violent, since this behavior increases risk of injury. In fact, the players should be told specifically not to make contact with one another. If athletes are involved in contact sports, the defensive player protecting the end zone can use blocking pads to increase sport specificity and to minimize risk of injury.

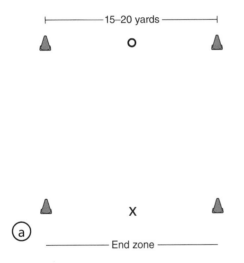

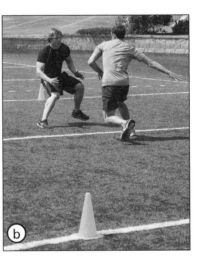

GAMES FOR IMPROVING QUICKNESS

Games that incorporate quickness skills are a fun way to increase athletes' motivation and enthusiasm for training. The quickness games in this section also help athletes develop their situational-movement skills and body awareness.

Red Light, Green Light

This drill improves quickness and teaches athletes how to effectively accelerate and decelerate. Two cones are placed 40 yards (37 m) apart. Athletes should stand by one cone and the coach should stand by the other. On the *green light* command, the athletes sprint forward as far as possible before the coach yells *red light!* On this command, the athletes immediately stop in place. When the coach calls *green light* again, the athletes resume sprinting toward the second cone. The coach continues to call out commands until an athlete passes the second cone.

```
├─────────────────────── 40 yards ───────────────────────┤
X
X
X
▲                                                    ▲ Coach
X
X
X
```

Knee Tag

This drill improves sport-specific speed and quickness for combative athletes. It also helps them learn to read and appropriately respond to their opponents' movements. Four cones or markers are set up in a square, with sides 6 feet (2 m) long. Two athletes stand approximately 3 feet (1 m) apart in the center of the square, face each other, and assume staggered stances. At the whistle, one athlete attempts to touch the opponent's knees (see photo). The opponent should dodge as needed to avoid being touched. The first athlete scores a point each time he tags the opponent's knees. Athletes should perform the game for approximately 15 to 30 seconds and then switch roles. The game can be repeated multiple times. However, athletes should rest for 30 to 60 seconds between bouts. After each athlete has had equal opportunities to score, the one who has earned the most points wins.

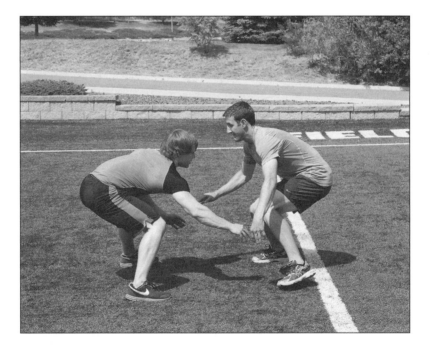

Heads or Tails

This game develops first-step quickness and improves reaction time. Two cones are placed 20 to 40 yards (18–37 m) apart, and another cone is placed halfway between them. At the center cone, two athletes face each other with their hands outstretched and their fingertips touching directly over the cone (photo *a*). The athletes then assume an athletic position, dropping their hands down to their sides. The coach designates one player as *heads* and the other as *tails*. The coach flips a coin and calls out which side of the coin is facing up. The designated athlete turns (photo *b*) and attempts to sprint past the cone originally behind him before being tagged by the other athlete (photo c). Points are given to any athlete who makes it to the scoring zone without being tagged or to any player who tags the fleeing runner outside of the designated safe area. Athletes should repeat the game 6 to 12 times.

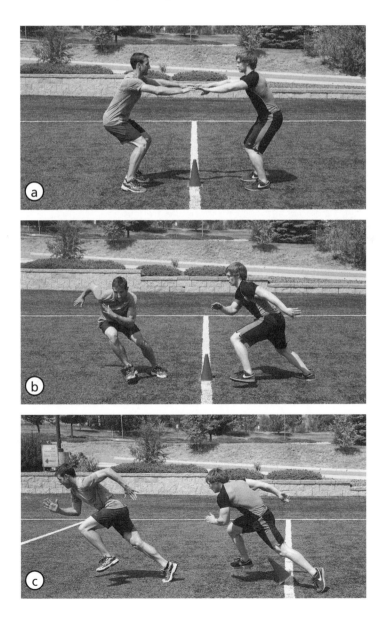

Sharks and Minnows

The purpose of this game is to improve situational awareness and to teach athletes to read an opponent's body movements. Four cones are set up to create a playing area that measures approximately 40 by 20 yards (37 by 18 m). One or two athletes assume the role of sharks (defensive players) and position themselves in the center of the playing area. The remaining players, or minnows (offensive players), line up on either end of the playing area. This game tends to work best with at least 6 minnows and no more than 20. The size of the playing area will largely determine the number of players. On command, the minnows attempt to sprint from one end of the playing area to the other without being tagged by the sharks. A minnow who is tagged by a shark switches roles with that player. Athletes should play this game for approximately 5 to 10 minutes.

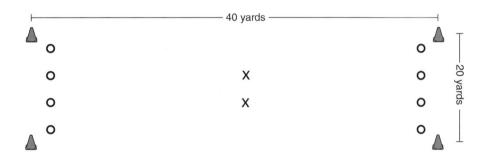

Everybody Is It

This game helps improve athletes' situational awareness and teaches them to read an opponent's body movements. Four cones are set up in a square, with sides approximately 15 to 20 yards (14–18 m) long. Three or four athletes should spread out over the designated playing area. On the *go* command, these athletes attempt to tag as many of the other players as possible without being tagged themselves. An athlete who is tagged must immediately perform a preassigned task or movement, such as five jumping jacks or push-ups, before returning to the game. If a dispute arises about which athlete was tagged first, both athletes must perform the assigned task. Athletes should play this game for 15 to 20 seconds, resting for 45 to 60 seconds between sets.

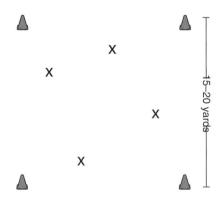

Twenty-One

This game improves quickness, situational awareness, and strategic thinking. It works best with two or three athletes. The game begins when the coach tosses a reaction ball into the air. (A reaction ball is a small rubberized ball that bounces in an unpredictable manner when thrown or tossed. See photo.) Players must allow the ball to bounce at least once before attempting to catch it. However, the player who catches the ball receives a point for each bounce of the ball prior to the catch. For example, if an athlete catches the ball after it has bounced twice, that player receives two points. The first athlete to accumulate 21 points wins the game.

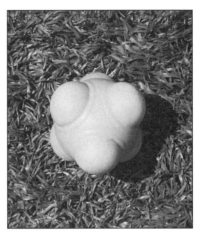

Team Keep-Away

This game improves quickness, situational awareness, and teamwork. Four cones are set up to create a playing area of 30 by 30 yards (27 m), which works well for a group of 8 to 10 athletes. For more players, the coach may double the length of the field. Athletes divide into two equal teams and spread out over the two halves of the playing area. The coach starts the game by blowing a whistle, starting a stopwatch, and passing a ball (of any kind) to one of the teams. The athletes in possession of the ball pass it among themselves while trying to prevent the other team from gaining possession. When an athlete gains possession of the ball, he must pass it within five seconds or automatically forfeit it to the opposing team. Athletes may grab, intercept, or strip the ball as necessary to gain possession. Play the game for a predetermined amount of time, usually one to three minutes. The team in possession of the ball when time runs out or the team that has the ball longest wins.

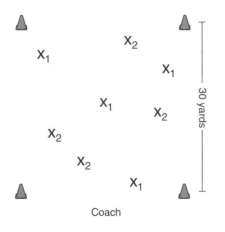

Ultimate

This game, a modified version of Ultimate Frisbee, is great for developing situational awareness and teamwork. Four cones are set up to create a playing area with sides about 50 yards (46 m) long. The rules to this game are similar to those of football. However, limited physical contact is allowed and the receiving athlete's role is slightly modified. Athletes should play this game in a large, open area at least the size of a basketball court. They may use different types of balls, such as basketballs and rugby balls. Athletes divide into two equal teams, and each team goes to its side of the playing area. One team begins the game as the offense and the other team begins as the defense.

The game starts when a designated athlete on the defensive team puts the ball in play by throwing it to the offensive team's side of the playing field. When an athlete on the offensive team catches or picks up the ball, he must remain stationary and throw the ball to another athlete on the team. This process is repeated to move the ball down the playing area toward the opponent's goal line. Teams score a point when one of their players crosses the opponent's goal line and catches the ball in the air. If a throw is intercepted or if a point is scored, then the defensive team becomes the offensive team.

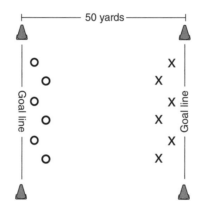

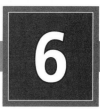

Agility and Quickness Program Design

Joel Raether
David J. Sandler

Without a plan, improving performance on the game field is like playing roulette—it is a game of chance. All training should have a purpose and a specific path toward achieving a goal.[35] Agility and quickness training is no exception. It is neither effective nor smart to randomly assign training drills in the hope that agility and quickness will improve. Therefore, athletes must progressively incorporate the proper exercises and drills into their training programs.

The exercises selected force specific adaptation, but other variables are also important, such as the environment, injury history, current training status, and recovery periods. Since no two athletes are alike, each one's ability will differ. Athletes should properly adjust drills and training sessions so that they can progress based on their own level of ability and proficiency. Although agility requires the ability to change direction while maintaining speed, the degree to which athletes need to work on specific agility skills will depend on individual strengths and weaknesses.[8, 25]

SAFETY CONSIDERATIONS

Safety must always be the first concern to ensure the optimal learning and training environment. This section discusses some basic safety recommendations that allow athletes to experience all the potential benefits of agility and quickness training.

Training Area

Agility drills require sufficient space for coaches and athletes to safely coexist and perform. For this reason, a barrier of at least 5 yards (5 m) around every side of the drill is recommended. Today, many facilities are designed so that agility training can be performed within the weight room. However, the more open space that is available for each drill, the easier and safer it will be to perform this type of training. As a general rule of thumb, coaches should allow approximately 40 to 50 square feet (12–15 m) of space per athlete.[22, 32]

Training Surface

In order to maximize agility training, the training surfaces should be similar to those of the actual competition. For example, since athletes play on both artificial turf and grass in sports such as soccer and football, they should train on both surfaces. Although it is important to be mindful of the training surfaces athletes will compete on, nonspecific training on alternative surfaces can help combat staleness and offer variety during the off-season or times of lower intensity.

Athlete Attire

In general, athletes should train in athletic shorts and a T-shirt. This allows a coach to see joint angles and to analyze posture and balance as athletes move through drills. On hot days, athletes may need additional shirts, since wet shirts do not effectively remove sweat and body heat. When performing sport-specific drills, athletes should ideally wear attire similar to competition gear. This helps them learn to move comfortably while wearing competition attire. The same rule applies to footwear. When they train, athletes should wear shoes similar to those they intend to wear during competition. For example, baseball players should wear the same cleats during practice and drills that they intend to wear during games. However, if they are performing agility and quickness drills indoors, turf or cross-training shoes may be more appropriate.

Injury Status and Orthopedic Issues

Every coach and most athletes must face the issue of evaluating injuries and training readiness at some point. Rehabilitation must aim to improve speed and quickness and bring the athlete back to game readiness as soon as possible. It should begin as soon as the athlete is medically cleared to do so. Athletes may delay starting a rehabilitation program after an injury, which can lengthen the amount of time needed to return to play. The coach should make the decision in conjunction with the medical personnel treating the athlete.

The rehabilitation program should progress from a basic level, increasing in intensity as the athlete demonstrates proficiency of pain-free movement. The athlete's time loss can be minimized if this process is initiated seamlessly with the sports medicine staff, strength and conditioning department, and the coaches.

Fatigue

The harder the work or intensity of training, the greater the level of fatigue the athlete will experience. Athletes must execute drills at full speed to achieve optimal results.[11] When fatigue sets in, technique often deteriorates. Athletes begin to perform movement patterns poorly. During speed training, coaches must watch athletes for faulty technique and signs of fatigue. If coaches observe a loss of good posture, improper positioning of the center of mass, or other technique flaws, they must take corrective measures and modify the training session.

Often, coaches require athletes to continue speed drills when they are overly fatigued. This essentially turns the session into conditioning, or metabolic-based, training. Conditioning and speed training are distinct types with different intensity levels. Therefore, they should not be performed simultaneously.[7, 14, 29, 30] Athletes must perform agility and quickness drills before doing conditioning drills. Coaches should create work-to-rest ratios that promote full recovery between sets. This allows athletes to maintain proper form and gamelike intensity during training sessions.

TRAINING INTENSITY AND VOLUME

Intensity is a measure of effort often compared to the maximum amount of weight that can be lifted or maximal movement speed. It is a major factor in determining the overall stress of a training session. During agility and quickness training, the speed of movement and power produced in each drill determines the degree of positive adaptations.[15, 17, 20] Athletes should perform all drills with maximum speed and power. Anything less decreases the force and power developed, minimizing the training's effect.

It can be hard to measure training intensity during agility and quickness training. However, coaches can accurately determine this by measuring the time athletes take to perform a drill or monitoring their training and recovery heart rates. Heart rate should spike in drills that last six seconds or longer. Over the duration of a training cycle, athletes should take less time to perform the same drill. This indicates an improvement in speed. From the standpoint of anaerobic endurance, if athletes' rest times decrease and their heart rates recover faster, they have made a positive gain through training.

Generally speaking, the volume of agility training can be classified by the number of sets performed, the length of time or distance required in drills, the amount of recovery provided per set, the frequency of training sessions, and the intensity (how quickly in time and the amplitudes of each movement) of the drills being performed.[9] This can be more aptly coined as the *volume load* of training stress induced.[31]

Keep in mind that time is directly influenced by intensity. So, if athletes perform drills maximally, speed should drop off quickly. Extending drill duration is counterproductive, turning speed training into a conditioning session. During a maximal effort, athletes can only maintain speed in agility or quickness drills for about seven seconds. Coaches may use drills that last longer to train endurance in the areas of speed or the anaerobic energy system, but these may not positively affect maximum change-of-direction speed. Typically, athletes perform drills for quickness, acceleration, or quick foot movements for three to five seconds.

Intensity and Volume by Drill Type

For line, ladder, and cone drills, the total number of sprints is determined by experience level and is measured as total work time. For example, if athletes perform five drills of 5 seconds each, the total work volume would be 25 seconds. Table 6.1 shows the total sprint volume for agility work for different experience levels. These standards and guidelines are very useful for athletes and coaches. They include a variety of drills and patterns for any agility or quickness program.

Coaches need to monitor volume and intensity, using drills to improve quickness and agility and not just to add a conditioning component to exercises. The training session can improve the specific areas needed to increase performance results for agility and quickness by setting up appropriate intensity levels, duration of drills, recovery periods, and volume of drills.

Dot drills are recorded by the number of single-foot contacts with the ground per session (not the number of contacts per exercise). For example, four sets of 10 reps with a type of movement that involves both feet would result in 80 repetitions. Table 6.2 provides volumes for varying levels of intensity. This table assumes that each movement is done at 100 percent effort. However, when attempting new drills, athletes should use slower speeds until they have mastered the technique. They may progress to full speed when they have demonstrated proficiency.

Table 6.1 Volume of Training Based on Experience Level

Experience level	Work volume per training session	Rest between drills*
Beginner	2 min.	30 sec.
Intermediate	3 min.	30–40 sec.
Advanced	4 min.	30–50 sec.

*As the number of drills increases, rest time should also increase if maximal speed is desired. The cumulative effect of fatigue plays a role in the breakdown of both technique and speed.

Table 6.2 Recommended Foot Contacts per Session

Level	Low-intensity drills	Moderate-intensity drills	High-intensity drills
Beginner	80	60	40
Intermediate	100	80	60
Advanced	140	120	100

Note that the rest periods between sets should not be shorter than two minutes unless the work period is very short. Rest periods shorter than two minutes limit the total amount of work that athletes can perform, decreasing the effectiveness of the training program. Very short rest periods do not allow for complete recovery of the ATP-CP energy system (see the following section for more information) or for the removal of lactic acid.

Power and Speed Drop-Offs

Agility training, like strength training, is planned using sets and repetitions. In strength training, the amount of resistance (or load) selected controls the workout's intensity. If 67 to 75 percent of athletes' one-repetition maximum is on the bar, they generally reach a failure point after 10 to 12 reps. Unlike strength training, athletes should never take sets of agility drills to the point of muscular failure. During agility training, they should base the duration of the set on decreases in power or speed of movement.

Physics defines *power* as the time rate of performing work.[21] More plainly, power is represented as the amount of work divided by the time needed to execute it. Additionally, work is equivalent to the force applied and distance that a given mass moves. All of these factors depend on energy. In this case, consider the amount of energy an athlete can exert in a task. The amount of energy that can be produced determines both the amount and duration of work.

During high-intensity agility activity, the body relies primarily on the ATP-CP, or the adenosine triphosphate and creatine phosphate, stored in the muscles for energy. The ATP-CP system is the most powerful energy system in the body, producing huge amounts of energy in a very short amount of time. Unfortunately, the supply of ATP-CP is limited. Activity quickly depletes the energy system, resulting in a drop in speed and power and a decrease in performance and technique. The rate of depletion of the ATP-CP system depends on the type of drill. It is generally limited to 3 to 15 seconds of continuous, all-out work.[36]

For this reason, if athletes experience a drop in speed of 10 percent from the best score obtained during a scheduled test session, it is best to discontinue agility training for that day. Determining a drop-off is both an art and a science that develops with time and experience. However, coaches and athletes should be aware of these signs that indicate fatigue is setting in and power is dropping off.

The most obvious sign of power drop-off is technique breakdown. Poor foot or body position, improper technique, inability to maintain balance, and general slowing down indicate that athletes should terminate a drill. Generally, the ability to effectively decelerate tends to fail first. Because of this, coaches should watch carefully as athletes attempt to decelerate during drill performance. If technique falters, looks awkward, or takes too long, coaches should extend rest times or terminate the drill.

A more straightforward approach is to simply time each repetition and compare it to the athlete's best performance. This may be difficult with larger groups, so coaches may prefer to use prior test results as a standard of performance. The advantage to this method is that coaches only have to calculate results once after the test session. It is quick and easy to administer to large groups of athletes. If coaches have each athlete's best score, they can determine fatigue rates just by glancing at their test scores.

Unfortunately, relying on test results doesn't allow for program adjustments as a result of performance between test sessions. If test results are the determining factor for increasing rest times or stopping a training session, retests should be scheduled routinely. Coaches should test each exercise that will be included in training. Whether the 10 percent drop is based on test results or on the best result for each training session, they should give a formal testing session every six to eight weeks to ensure the program is delivering the desired results.

EXERCISE AND DRILL SELECTION

Building a house requires certain tools. The same is true when trying to build an athlete. Selecting the best tools for the job helps coaches and athletes achieve their goals quickly and efficiently. However, if they choose the wrong tools for the job, it will take them longer to achieve their goals. In some cases, this choice may make it impossible to reach these goals. These guidelines, along with the information from other chapters, allow coaches to develop a progressive program and an effective training schedule. Coaches should consider the unique situation of each athlete and take the time to lay out a proper program for attaining goals. This will ensure that they have the right tools in their toolbox to get the job done.

Specificity of Training

Selecting appropriate exercises and drills is a key design component of agility and quickness programs. When choosing or designing drills, consider the concepts of specificity and transfer of training. Specificity of training has a variety of meanings and can be applied to energy systems, movement patterns, and speed of movement. In simplest terms, *specificity* means training for the particular demands of the sport by simulating all or parts of the performance during a training session.[10] The concept of specificity is based on *transfer of training,* which refers to the amount of fitness improvement that carries over to competition.

Proponents of specificity believe that the more closely athletes simulate a sport movement, the greater the transfer of training will be. Ample evidence (both anecdotal and in motor-learning literature) supports this notion.[9, 19, 27, 28, 34] Consider tennis players who take up squash. They will be relatively successful the first time they play the new sport because the movements used in tennis are close enough to those used in squash for a high level of transfer to occur. This is not to say that the tennis player will become a top squash player, but it does highlight the idea that athletes can effect improvement by training movement patterns that are closely related to those of their sports.

Agility drills teach the brain how to control the body when reacting to a stimulus. By focusing on specific cues, agility drills help improve and correct body position, balance, coordination, and explosive movement patterns that are executed in competition. Quickness drills and acceleration within agility patterns improve intermuscular and intramuscular coordination.[18] Additionally, incorporating drills that reflect similar movements of a specific sport appear to elicit positive correlations for optimal transfer.[9] In other words, if a sport requires lateral body movements, the athlete should perform agility drills that specifically address lateral movement patterns.[9]

The degree of specificity used when designing drills depends on the athlete's competitive level, age, fitness level, body control, and athleticism.[9] The following drill progression helps maximize transfer of training and sport-specific agility performance.

1. Drills for General Footwork and Body Position

The starting point for all agility work is good body control and mechanics. The first drill level teaches forward, backward, and lateral movement skills, including starts, stops, turns, corners, and cuts. This phase of development is coaching intensive. Frequent feedback and correction with regard to biomechanics are essential if athletes are to get full value from the more complex drills in later stages.

2. Drills for Sport-Specific Footwork and Body Position

Although many sports share common basic movement patterns, the use of implements like racquets and balls can cause changes in body position that affect balance, quickness, and ability to change direction. For instance, coaches often incorporate a vigorous forward and backward arm swing similar to that used in sprinting into a basic ladder drill. This can be a great drill for developing basic movement skills, but the arm action may be of little benefit to a lacrosse player who holds a stick in both hands. These players may perform the same drill while holding a stick to learn the balance and body positioning required on the field.

3. External Reaction Drills

The term *agility* is often used synonymously with change-of-direction speed, athleticism, and sport speed.[9, 11, 21, 23, 24] Although the ability to change direction is definitely part of the equation, agility is much more than these definitions. It encompasses perceptual factors, such as the ability to anticipate and react to a stimulus, to select the appropriate movement and direction, and to make necessary body adjustments to optimize stride rate and frequency.

Visual- and auditory-reaction components may help athletes further develop decision-making skills and learn basic and sport-specific patterns of body position and footwork. When first introducing drills with an additional external stimulus, coaches may emphasize general body position and footwork drills until athletes demonstrate command of movements. Next, they can move on to sport-specific footwork and body-position drills with external stimuli.

4. Skilled Agility Drills

Designing good skilled agility drills requires a higher level of knowledge of the sport and more thought, imagination, and planning than other forms of agility training do. Some distinct performance advantages of skilled agility drills include the following:

▶ Skilled agility training can be more time efficient, allowing athletes to train for both skill and fitness simultaneously. This can be a big advantage in high school or club sport programs with limited gym, field, or ice time.

▶ The strength and conditioning coach has more control over the athlete's total training volume. Very often the work done in practice is not counted in the overall training volume when conditioning programs are designed. Traditionally, the strength and conditioning coach has little or no control over the type and intensity of work done in practice. As a result, many athletes show up for training sessions already fatigued. This makes agility sessions less effective.

▶ Skilled agility training can use games and gamelike situations to create a competitive environment that motivates athletes to train at a higher level of intensity than they normally would.

▶ Athletes learn to use sport-specific perceptual cues to improve their reactions and agility performances.

Motor Development Approach

The term *sport specific* is often used to describe how a particular exercise or movement pattern mimics the patterns performed during athletic competition.[29] To maximize the transfer-of-training effect and improve neuromuscular coordination, coaches often try to duplicate movement patterns during training that occur in competition. However, agility training should initially focus on improving overall coordination, balance, and ability to change direction by using patterned learning that reinforces fast, precise motor recruitment to enhance movement control.[9, 13, 23, 33] Next, training should progress to drills that aid in the development of sport-specific kinesthetic awareness and the ability to quickly change direction with control within the sporting context. Essentially, athletes should develop good general skills before developing sport-specific agility and quickness. This will help ensure that they have a good base to work from to enhance their future sport-specific development.

The motor skills that are paramount for success include heightened internal processing of external information (i.e., a defender, ball, goal, and so on) and the ability of the central nervous system to improve neuromuscular efficiency to complete the desired task.[34] If athletes can improve their body position, maintain their center of balance, and move quickly in the intended direction, they will improve their opportunities for success. This is achieved through the complex processing of sensory information. Athletes must figure out a plan and send that information to the muscles in a precise way so that they can execute the movement properly.[25] Neural processing occurs within 200 milliseconds in most athletic endeavors.[26, 27] Athletes develop these skills through repetitive practice.

As athletes continue to practice specific drills, their ability to reproduce the exact movement patterns with speed and accuracy improves.[34] During the execution of the drill, they must emphasize good body position and proper mechanics while increasing speed. Since no two plays are ever identical in sports, drills need to progress in difficulty and variety by requiring quicker and sharper directional changes, variable movement patterns that maintain athletic specificity, and the incorporation of a reactionary component when athletes are ready.[33]

Athletes should train specific movement patterns before working on the ability to transition smoothly from one movement pattern to the next (e.g., backpedal to a forward sprint). Drills should include all of the movements that occur in the chosen sport, such as shuffling, backpedaling, sharp cutting in all directions, and taking crossover steps. When athletes demonstrate proficiency with basic movements, coaches may add random and reactionary types of stimuli that are visual, audible, and tactile to complete the training. Essentially, the goal is to progress through a continuum of processing information, enhancing athletes' motor programming and helping them reach a level of automatization.[9, 24]

Whole Versus Part Learning

Several schools of thought exist about how to teach a movement, practice a skill, and design drills that emulate specific movement patterns. Much of this decision relies on the initial movement ability of the person trying to perform the drills. Advanced athletes usually exhibit better balance, speed, and body control than beginners do. Although some athletes tend to have natural talents, many need to learn a drill or movement step by step in order to be proficient. This means that during agility training, athletes should learn the basic parts of each skill before progressing to the full drill or target movement.[26] As a result, athletes should first learn basic step patterns (such as shuffling and backpedaling), basic transfers of body position (such as cutting), and how to maintain balance during motion.

To that end, drills should focus on the individual movements (or discrete tasks) that make up partial skills. Next, those skills will come together to make up the full drill (or a serial task).[9, 24] The better athletes are at these basic skills, the greater the likelihood that they will be able to transfer that training to on-field performance. For instance, if athletes do not shuffle correctly, drills that require shuffling will be of minimal value to them. Instead, coaches should emphasize correct shuffling before athletes more on to a more advanced drill that combines several discrete tasks or movements. This is especially true when it comes to making cuts and maintaining good body position. If athletes cannot cut properly, they will become less and less effective in their movement patterns as drills continue to increase in difficulty.

A beginning athlete may need to focus on simple drills and basic movement skills for several weeks before progressing to more complex drills. The temptation to increase drill complexity and rapidly progress athletes from basic to advanced training generally stems from the desire to reduce boredom from repetitive practice. If basketball players take thousands of shots from the free throw line to reinforce motor pathways, they should be able to perform thousands of repetitions of basic movements in agility drills.

Blocked Versus Random Practice

As previously discussed, most athletes improve at drill performance relatively quickly. Blocked drills improve specific skills, such as transitions, footwork, or body position. The pattern or course is predetermined so that the athlete knows exactly how the drill will be performed. This blocked practice creates the basis for the neural pattern by teaching the body how to maintain position when changing direction or performing movement skills. The skill sets are learned and are ready to be used as required.[27, 28]

Most sports are random in nature, which makes both drill selection and continuous training quite difficult. Every time a quarterback throws a pass, it varies in speed, angle, and placement. The opponent must react in an unexpected manner or pattern to successfully make a play that varies constantly. For that reason, coaches must introduce open drills in which the movement patterns are not predetermined.[12] Once athletes become proficient at the basic skills and transitions, coaches should increase the difficulty in order to prepare them for the unknown.

Drills that are open in nature and have a reactionary component teach athletes how to maintain correct movement patterns and body position while reacting to unknown stimuli. During training, the reaction stimulus should be visual, audible, or tactile (based on the concept of specificity). However, it should also be precise, so that the athlete has enough time to receive and interpret the stimulus and develop a movement pattern to correctly perform the drill.

The drills should be progressive in nature, first starting with reactionary stimuli that are easy to process, and then increasing in difficulty. For example, if athletes are to cut on a visual cue, the coach can initially give them ample time to react, and then gradually reduce the amount of time athletes have to react as they improve. In fact, perceptual reactionary training has been shown to improve athletes' game awareness and decision-making ability.[1, 2, 4, 5, 6, 15, 16, 17, 20] Moreover, it increases anticipatory skills in sport.[3] The importance of progression, which allows athletes time to learn to react in shorter and shorter time frames while maintaining correct movement patterns and body position, cannot be overemphasized.

CHAPTER 7

Sport-Specific Agility and Quickness Training

This chapter discusses agility and quickness training and drills for specific sports (see table 7.1 for more information). Keep in mind that each section author and the book editors selected some of their favorite drills for the featured sports. Although these are definitely not the only drills that can be used for a particular sport-training program, they provide some general suggestions and considerations for developing a comprehensive training program.

Athletes can easily adapt these drills or substitute others from chapters 4 and 5 based on their level of performance, training background, yearly training cycle, and training goals. These drills, along with those from chapters 4 and 5, make up a sample program that is meant to give coaches and athletes ideas for agility training. Athletes can implement a variety of other drills in their place. As time progresses, they will be able to come up with drills that are best suited for their particular sport. The rate of progression should be determined by the athletes' ability to complete the correct pattern or movement, as well as by their physiological abilities, such as strength. Coaches should base progression on athletes' body control, awareness, speed of movement, and technique when performing an activity or drill.

Table 7.1 Sport-Specific Training for Agility and Quickness

Sport	Page number
Baseball and softball	128
Basketball	131
Football	136
Ice hockey	139
Lacrosse	141
Soccer	144
Tennis	151
Volleyball	153
Wrestling	157

BASEBALL AND SOFTBALL

Javair Gillett

Baseball and softball require a unique combination of athletic skills. Better athletes in these sports can maintain balance and control during situations that call for unrehearsed, rapid decision making. This consistency often makes even the most difficult plays look easy. Agility and quickness training on and off the field improves baseball and softball players' mobility, coordination, and reaction time. The combination of these improved movement skills maximizes their power output and speed potential.

A complete routine, performed daily, creates the readiness athletes' bodies need to compete at their highest potential day in and day out. This approach is both mental and physical. Forms of agility training are applied daily on the field during games and practices, but coaches should always remember that developing a complete athlete and, ultimately, creating a better and healthier player requires additional training. Coaches should incorporate athletic movement drills in all practice sessions and pregame routines.

Agility requires proprioception for the proper mechanical positioning of a joint. With this understanding, the purpose of agility exercises and drills is to improve athletes' neuromuscular communication and coordination while executing dynamic movements on the field. Therefore, they don't perform agility drills solely to develop quick and explosive movements, but more important, to improve the speed of communication between the central nervous system and the musculoskeletal system. In other words, a properly designed agility-training program may help reduce the time it takes for the brain to send a signal to the muscle through the body's neural pathways to trigger a preferred response, thus improving overall quickness.

Baseball and softball players can improve agility and quickness in several ways. For this reason, agility training can be classified into three categories:

1. *Range of motion.* Proper movement should be pain free, using the soft and connective tissues that surround and support the joints.

2. *Movement technique.* Efficient awareness and joint positioning must take place to optimize the use of these tissues.

3. *Reactivity.* This is the central nervous system's instantaneous ability to respond, to communicate this response to the rest of the body, and to coordinate a desired action.

Agility exercises and drills focus on acquiring adequate range of motion in the joints, positioning joints more efficiently, and improving reaction time to elicit results that are more forceful, more powerful, and faster.[6] The actual intensity (the resistance used, the difficulty level of the exercise, and the speed) at which the drills are performed often depends on an athlete's current level of training, goals, age, motor skill acquisition, past and current injuries, as well as other controllable and uncontrollable factors.

Injured athletes, novices, and youths may not have developed the motor skills they need to place their joints in correct positions. As a result, they must first learn, or relearn, proper joint positioning. Even the simplest changes in movement can lead to impressive results in total athletic performance on the field. Athletes can modify programs to fit their needs and goals by adjusting the intensity of exercises or drills.

TAILORING TRAINING TO INDIVIDUAL ATHLETES

Due to differences in athletes' ages, athletic abilities, and conditioning levels, a coach must always be able to make adjustments to a training program within a team setting. Young athletes and beginners should use a combination of exercises, starting with still positions and moving at slow speeds to learn the correct joint positions and which muscles are used to perform each task. This basic body awareness is still trained at the highest levels.

Nevertheless, all athletes who enter a baseball or softball game will be required to perform skills at high rates of speed, whether they are able to perform them well or not. Therefore, to prepare for game-speed situations, coaches should utilize the most basic drills that address the demands of all aspects of the game. Prescribed movements should begin slowly with a good dynamic warm-up, and then move into more explosive exercises and drills. Athletes should perform two sets of each drill featured in the dynamic warm-up section in chapter 4.

Of course, in a game, the perfect situation is not always present. The body is asked to respond to abnormal tasks (i.e., fielding a bunt and throwing from one leg). As a result, an effective agility and quickness program involves intricate knowledge of the game, movements that are called for on the field, and purposeful exercises to adapt to these demands. As a result, more advanced athletes need to learn how to position their bodies properly in multiple directions at multiple joint angles. Agility training on one leg, such as when performing single-leg hops in and out of a ladder, can offer a more difficult setting for athletes to improve body control and make quick adjustments to unpracticed situations.

PROGRAM DESIGN

When coaching large groups, splitting a team into smaller agility stations for performing different drills with a specific focus makes training sessions easier to organize and allows players to maximize their training time. To maintain management and organization, one player in each group can perform a drill while the other group members rest and wait their turn. Once the entire group has performed the drill, each group will rotate to the next station. The following example describes how these stations can be organized.

Team Agility Drill

Coaches should divide players equally among four stations (e.g., for 20 players, 5 athletes would be at each station). Athletes complete two exercises per station using 10-second sets for each exercise or drill. After each player in a group has performed both exercises, the group rotates to the next station.

Station 1: Range of Motion

Choose two of the dynamic warm-up drills from chapter 4 (starting on page 56).

Station 2: Movement Technique

1. *High-knee run and backpedal* (pages 60 and 77). The athlete runs 5 yards (5 m) with good high-knee technique. At the 5-yard mark, the athlete turns 180 degrees and backpedals for an additional 5 yards.
2. *90-degree rounds or cuts* (pages 82 and 83).

Station 3: Reactivity

1. *Forward and backward hops* (ladder drill used for body control; variation of the drill on page 62). With both feet slightly closer together than shoulder width and with shoulders parallel with the ladder rungs, the athlete stands at the end of the ladder and hops into each box. This movement can be done moving forward or backward.
2. *Ickey shuffle* (ladder drill used for foot quickness; see page 68).

Station 4: Movement Patterns and Skills Specific to Baseball and Softball

1. *Lateral shuffle* (page 77). The athlete should throw backhand across the body.
2. *Forward run* (page 77). The athlete should practice multiangle ball pickups.

BASKETBALL

Al Biancani

Basketball requires athletes to move forward, backward, laterally, and diagonally. Players also need to change directions in a split second, go from full speed to a standstill, and move from standing to full speed quickly. Defensive players must be able to stay with the people they are guarding as well as go around and under picks as quickly as possible. On offense, athletes need to dribble and try to get past their opponents. The person without the ball must run and cut to get open to either get a shot or to pass. Quick foot movement is imperative for success in basketball. For this reason, all of these abilities have a definite and profound effect on success in a game situation.

MOVEMENT DRILLS WITH A BALL

When performing any of the cone drills featured in this book, dribbling a ball assists players in perfecting movement patterns and adds an element of sport specificity. These combinations of cone drills and other quickness exercises are a great warm-up that can lead into more complex agility drills. Coaches can change patterns and movements to increase the level of difficulty, since these require more technical mastery to perform. They can modify any of these drills to be more specific to basketball by incorporating the following movements and variations while using a ball.

- ▶ *Crossover.* When cutting from a cone, the athlete uses a crossover dribble to add sport specificity.
- ▶ *Spin.* When making a cut at a cone, the athlete uses a spin move to transition into another change of direction.
- ▶ *In and out.* The athlete drives toward the cone with a hard dribble. At the cone, he stops, decelerates, and backs away from it. The athlete moves forward to the next cone and repeats the movement pattern.
- ▶ *Between the legs.* When changing direction at a cone to move to the next one, the athlete dribbles the ball between the legs.
- ▶ *Behind the back.* This is similar to between the legs except that the athlete changes direction and takes the ball behind the back to change ball movement and hand placement.
- ▶ *Into a double-team and out.* This is similar to the in and out drill. Here, the player needs to backpedal with more steps to practice the movement needed to get out of a double-team situation, which occurs in games.

IN-THE-PAINT DRILLS

These drills are good for working in a small space. They require high amounts of activity *in the paint,* or around the basket. Coaches can modify traditional cone drills to create a variety of in-the-paint drills.

Diagonal Lateral Shuffle

Cone 1 is set up at one end of the free throw line and cone 2 is placed at the other end. The coach should places 10 rolls of tape along the cone 2 side of the lane, next to the painted line. The athlete starts at cone 1 and then shuffles to the first roll of tape and picks up the roll with the outside hand. While shuffling back to cone 1, he moves the tape into the other hand. The athlete places the tape near cone 1, and continues to shuffle to and from each of the other rolls of tape until he has transferred all the rolls to the area by cone 1. Beginners should perform this drill for no more than 12 seconds to avoid making the exercise a conditioning drill. The

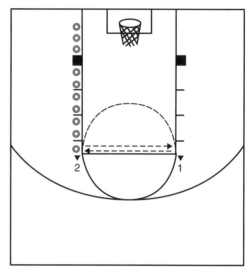

athlete should perform 5 sets and then build to 7 to 10 sets. Minimum rest periods of 30 seconds should be used with this drill. However, if form and technique suffer in subsequent sets, the rest periods can be increases to one or two minutes between sets.

Four Corners Drill

This drill is performed as discussed in chapter 4 on page 86. For this version, athletes dribble a ball for greater sport specificity. The athlete should start with 5 repetitions in each direction and build to 10.

X Drill

This drill is performed as discussed in chapter 4 on page 88. For this version, athletes dribble a ball for greater sport specificity. The athlete should start with 5 repetitions in each direction and build to 10.

Five-Cone Drills

These drills use the five-cone set-up pattern described in chapter 4 on page 89. Coaches may modify the distance between cones to challenge players in slightly different ways. Larger distances require less rapid changes of direction than smaller distances do, so athletes can use boxes of different sizes. Cones are placed in the shape of a box. The large box should have sides 10 yards (9 m) long, and the smaller box should have sides 5 yards (5 m) long. Athletes should go both ways through the boxes to ensure balanced training. Individual athletes can perform these drills for time. To add a bit of competition, coaches can set up two patterns for players to perform simultaneously for the best time. When athletes perform these drills, coaches should emphasize the following:

- Athletes must go around each cone, making sharp, crisp cuts.
- Athletes must use proper technique.
- Athletes must use quick foot movement.
- As they become proficient, athletes should perform all drills while dribbling a basketball for sport specificity.
- Athletes should start with the large box. When they are proficient at each drill, they should use the small box. The small box is useful when athletes are peaking for the season because most movement on the court occurs in a small space.

ADDITIONAL DRILLS

The following drills can be used alone as independent drills or in circuit training stations. These drills could also be used in combination with the In-the-Paint series of drills. The activities listed in the Twelve-Station Agility Circuit can be substituted with other activities to change up the circuit when needed.

Offense and Defense

This drill is a variation of the containment drill discussed in chapter 5 (page 108). It is great for working on defensive skills and dribbling movements. Two cones are set up four or five paces apart. Two players face each other at cone 1. Using different dribbles, the offensive player works to get by the opponent and reach cone 2. The defensive player points his nose at the offensive player's chest, keeps the hands up, and maintains a good defensive stance at all times. Once both players get to the opposite cone, they switch roles and continue. Players can do this drill back and forth 10 times. Timed sessions (up to two minutes per set) can also be used.

Twelve-Station Agility Circuit

This drill allows multiple athletes to train simultaneously. Athletes should start with two sets of 30 seconds per station before moving to the next station. They should build to 60 seconds per set. The rest period between sets and station changes should be at least 30 seconds long. Athletes should do all activities at full speed.

Station 1: Reverse Layup

A cone is placed on either side of the paint at a 45-degree angle to the basket and in a position 5 to 7 yards (5–6 m) back from the basket. The athlete starts at cone 1 with a ball. He touches cone 1, does a reverse pivot, dribbles to the basket, and does a reverse layup. After getting the rebound, the athlete sprints to cone 2, touches the cone, does a reverse pivot, dribbles to the basket, and does a reverse layup on the other side. The athlete repeats this movement for the designated duration of time.

Station 2: *X* in the Paint

For this drill, athletes perform various movements in an *X* pattern in the paint while dribbling a basketball. For example, a player starts in the corner of the lane at the free throw line, dribbles at a diagonal to the corner of the paint below the basket, then backpedals while dribbling to the other corner at the free throw line, and finishes by dribbling forward to the other corner under the basket.

Station 3: Shuffle and Wall Pass

Two cones are placed 5 to 10 feet (1.5–3 m) apart to form a line that is parallel to and 5 to 10 feet away from a wall. The athlete quickly shuffles back and forth between the two cones while doing different passes against the wall. Some options include chest passes, bounce passes, and overhead passes. The athlete must catch the ball and pass it again while moving laterally.

Station 4: Line and Dot Drills

Any of the line drills (page 62–64) and dot drills (page 75–76) from chapter 4 are good for foot quickness. As athletes gain proficiency, they can add different, more complex combinations of foot patterns. Furthermore, as players gain efficiency with each pattern, speed of foot movement is critical.

Station 5: Two-Cone Dunk

This station is the same as the one for the reverse layup, but the player must attempt to dunk a basketball or a lightweight medicine ball.

Station 6: Ladder With a Dribble

The athlete begins on one side of a speed-and-agility ladder, then does different foot patterns while dribbling the ball along the length of the ladder. The athlete should perform these drills both forward and backward.

Station 7: Hurdle Side Run

Two cones are placed 6 to 7 yards (5–6 m) apart. Between the cones, eight 3-inch (8 cm) or 5-inch (13 cm) hurdles are placed 2 feet (60 cm) apart, with the hurdles facing the cones. To start the drill, the athlete runs laterally over the hurdles while dribbling the ball. When he gets to the end, he changes hands and dribbles the other direction. As the athlete goes left, he uses the right hand; as he goes right, he uses the left hand.

Hurdle side run setup.

Station 8: Five-Cone Drill

Five cones are placed in the shape of a square, with one in the middle. The sides of the square should be 5 yards (5 m) long. The athlete performs various agility patterns, including slides, forward runs, backward runs, and so on. Each drill should be performed in both directions for balanced training.

Station 9: Cone Sprint With Dribble

 Eight cones are placed in a straight line with approximately 4 feet (120 cm) between each cone. The athlete weaves through the cones, sprinting while dribbling. When the athlete gets to the end of the cones, he does a reverse pivot and weaves back through the pattern, returning to the starting line. The player should alternate dribbling with both hands at this station.

Station 10: Zigzag Cones With Dribble

Five cones are placed in a zigzag pattern, with 3 feet (1 m) between cones. The athlete should perform a variety of dribbling patterns through the cones. When he gets to the last cone, he performs a rip move by dropping the shoulder and lowering the hips to get by the cone. Then, with a pivot, he turns with the ball and returns back through the pattern to the start.

Station 11: Slides in the Paint

This drill is a variation of the diagonal lateral shuffle; the setup is the same. For this version, the athlete moves to each cone by completing three slides across the lane, picking up a tape roll, completing three slides back across the lane while passing the roll to the other hand, and placing it on the floor on the starting side. The athlete moves to the remaining tape rolls in the manner of the coach's or athlete's choosing (examples include randomly, diagonally, or straight across). The player continues until the designated time, which is set specifically for each athlete, has lapsed.

Station 12: Jab Step, Crossover, and Jump Shot

One end of a heavy tube is attached around a sturdy pole, and the other is tied around the athlete's waist, toward his back. Tension on the tubing is essential. To start the drill, the athlete takes a jab step to the right, does a crossover dribble, steps to the left, and goes into a jump shot. The athlete then steps back and repeats this movement in the other direction. This drill should be done on the court if possible. If the needed equipment is not available for court use, it can be done in a training facility. In this case, the athlete should go through the motions of a proper jump shot.

FOOTBALL

Todd Durkin

Superior agility and quickness are clear discriminating factors among football players at all levels. These skills improve performance, decrease risk of injury, and improve evasiveness by allowing athletes to fake or neutralize an opponent.[30] Although many drills work on overall agility, quickness, and evasiveness, coaches can create position-specific drills by combining closed and open drills in a random order for a more chaotic environment. Athletes who can execute these drills successfully should be best prepared to react during competition.[8, 31] Football requires a diversity of movement skills that are based on positional requirements. For purposes of simplicity, the positions can be broken down into three main categories.

INTERIOR LINE

The interior line includes the offensive line, defensive line, and the defensive ends. Areas of emphasis for these athletes include great explosion, acceleration, and balance. These athletes must also possess the skills to drop the hips within the base immediately and stay on their feet without getting knocked off course. Balance, center of gravity, and leverage play an important role with interior linemen. As always, base of support and foot quickness along with strength and power are also critical to success.[25, 31]

COMBO ATHLETES

Combo athletes include linebackers, tight ends, fullbacks, and safeties. Athletes who fall within this category must possess the size and power to deal with interior lineman, who are often larger, as well as the movement skills to react and compete with the skill or speed players. These players really need to integrate movement training throughout their programs. Although these athletes should focus on strength and hypertrophy, these skills should never come at the expense of speed, agility, and quickness. Tight ends and fullbacks must be able to block oncoming lineman and linebackers. They must also be able to apply skills, such as acceleration, deceleration, power cuts, speed cuts, and spin turns. Linebackers and safeties need first-step quickness, explosive power, and the ability to run forward, backward, and laterally. They must also be able to drop step to open the hips so that they can fall back into coverage using crossover and backpedal steps.[25, 31]

SKILL AND SPEED ATHLETES

Skill and speed athletes include wide receivers, running backs, defensive backs and corners, and quarterbacks. These athletes tend to operate in the open field more frequently. Wide receivers have the advantage of being able to master preprogrammed (closed) routes and vary them based on their opponents' defense and options within that play. Wide receivers must be able to cut at full speed in all directions. They often rely heavily on cutting on the inside leg at angles less than 90 degrees. They should also be proficient in power cuts, which primarily use the outside foot to redirect at an angle greater than 90 degrees.

Cornerbacks also need the keen ability to react to a fast-cutting wideout and a ball traveling at them at a high rate of speed. They function primarily in an open-skill environment and must react extremely quickly to the wide receiver's route and to the ball coming at them. Coordination is critical for cornerbacks.[31]

Footwork, quickness, and agility are pivotal for a quarterback as well. A drop back is a closed-skill drill. It can quickly become an open-skill drill with the onset of an oncoming defensive lineman or linebacker. Quarterbacks must work on their crossover ability, backpedaling, acceleration, deceleration, and setting up quickly in the pocket. Although many people think that a strong arm is the most important aspect of being a successful quarterback, foot speed, base of support, and leg and core strength also play an important role in the player's physical ability to compete.

All skill players use key movements, such as acceleration, deceleration, backpedaling, drops, and crossover runs. All of these players should master both general and special skills as well as closed-skill and open-skill movements. By incorporating various agility and quickness drills into the overall program, athletes will develop the evasiveness, quickness, and ability to enhance overall prowess on the gridiron.

DRILLS AND TIPS

Football coaches and athletes can use a variety of drills from chapter 4. Some recommendations for using the different types of drills follow. The setup of the drills (distance travelled, duration, and so on) determines the degree of specificity for each position.

▶ *Line drills.* Performing any of the lateral line drills in chapter 4 are great for improving transitions on the field. Coaches can vary the distance and movement patterns to make them position specific.

▶ *Ladder drills.* Coaches may vary the movement patterns, distance, and variety based on athletes' skill levels and positions.

▶ *Dot drills.* Coaches may vary the movement patterns and add stimuli, based on the athletes' ability and the movement progression.

▶ *Cone drills.* Coaches should use a variety of patterns. They can change the number of cones and the distances for each drill to match the skills of the athletes.

▶ *Specific agility drills.* The pro-agility drill, *T* drill, and combinations of other patterns and movements are useful for football.

Keep the following tips in mind when training agility and quickness for football athletes:

▶ To be quicker, athletes must learn how to stop. Deceleration is a major contributor for improving overall agility and quickness. The faster players can stop, the sooner they can start again. This also helps prevent injuries, such as hamstring strains.[24]

▶ Agility training should focus on reducing or minimizing the time between the eccentric and concentric action of a movement. Doing so allows athletes to produce the required force in the shortest amount of time.[30]

▶ Athletes must use an overall strength and conditioning approach to become quicker. To maximize results, players must have efficiency of movement, which involves coordination, dynamic balance, proprioception, and flexibility, in addition to overall body strength and power.

▶ Any muscle imbalances in strength or flexibility ultimately impede agility, quickness, and overall performance. Likewise, muscle imbalance can lead to injury.[31]

▶ Athletes should perform agility and quickness drills early in the routine when the nervous system is still fresh. The movement portion of the program can be incorporated right into the warm-up or can be done immediately after a 10- to 15-minute routine that includes a dynamic warm-up and joint-integrity drills.

▶ Athletes should focus on performing agility and quickness drills for quality, not just pure volume.

ICE HOCKEY

Katie Krall

Ice hockey is a game of speed, quickness, and agility. It is played on an ice sheet no bigger than 100 by 200 feet (30 by 60 m).[3] Although games are 60 minutes long, players typically perform high-intensity work for approximately 15 to 20 minutes in total during competition. On average, players rotate in shifts that last 30 to 45 seconds, resting for 3 to 4 minutes in between.[23] These shifts are anaerobic in nature, and include short, intense bursts of speed, as well as acceleration and abrupt changes of direction.[20] Ultimately, the ability to rapidly change direction in order to evade opponents and manipulate the flow of the game is advantageous.[9]

Agility and quickness training for hockey involves a high level of neuromuscular control and explosive power. Therefore, in order to fully maximize training adaptations, agility and quickness drills should be performed when the body is fully recovered.[20] Along with speed and power, several other components that are essential to improving agility and quickness are proper technique, posture, footwork, and balance.[33] Drills that mimic the specificity of hockey must address the constant variations in velocity that coordinate the timing of acceleration and deceleration. Athletes should rest adequately between bouts during practice in order to perform at full capacity and with proper technique. These intervals simulate the work-to-rest ratio experienced during competition, which is typically 1:4.[2]

Agility refers to the ability to coordinate sports-specific movements quickly while maintaining body control. *Quickness* refers to the ability to do these sport-specific movements as fast as possible with control. The initial response to agility training is primarily neural. However, performing numerous repetitions that focus on proper technique helps athletes ingrain neuromuscular patterns and improve strength and power.[2] As chapter 5 discusses, coaches can make agility drills more complex by progressing athletes from preprogrammed, closed-training drills to semicontrolled, open-training drills. The demands involved in hockey require athletes to maintain visual and auditory awareness while constantly processing new information. Therefore, to tailor these drills for the sport, coaches should incorporate cognitive stress while simultaneously tasking the athlete to complete a given agility pattern. Consequently, they should introduce a maximum of two or three external cues in advanced drills.

A training program geared specifically toward ice hockey must incorporate all planes of movements. This physically demanding sport requires athletes to maintain strength, power, agility, and balance throughout the duration of the game. Agility and quickness are inherent components of the sport that enable players to pursue or evade opponents as well as to react to the movement of the puck. These skills ultimately translate into enhanced performance. As players become more technically proficient, coaches should introduce external stimuli into agility training to further emulate the unpredictable nature of this sport.

LINE, LADDER, AND DOT DRILLS

Line drills, ladder drills for speed and agility, and dot drills enhance kinesthetic sense, full-body coordination, and foot speed. To perform them successfully, athletes must maintain good body control and execute the task accurately. Additionally, practicing these agility drills improves fundamental neuromuscular patterns, which are inherent to efficiently changing direction. Coaches should begin all of these drills at a very basic level and then progress to more complex drills according to the athlete's proficiency.

CONE DRILLS

Cones can be used to increase the number of times the athlete is required to change direction and to add more sport specificity to an agility and quickness program. The two- and three-cone drill combinations featured in chapter 4 are excellent for working on overall quality of movement and technique mastery. In addition, the star drill, attack and retreat drill, *T* drill, and pro-agility drill are excellent for improving change-of-direction speed. Furthermore, coaches can make sport-specific modifications to several of these drills. For example, to make the pro-agility drill more specific to hockey, the athlete can touch each line with the foot, rather than the hand, since placing a hand on the ice is neither required by the demands of the sport nor recommended for safety reasons. As with most agility drills, once the athlete has efficiently achieved high quality of movement, coaches can introduce auditory and visual cues to increase the complexity.

QUICKNESS DRILLS

In keeping with the ever-changing flow of ice hockey, athletes must quickly respond to a variety of stimuli. Responses include starting, stopping, and changing direction quickly. Open drills that require athletes to respond rapidly to auditory and visual cues improve first-step speed and provide a cognitive component that is specific to the sport. The ball drops (page 97) and quickness box drills (page 100) from chapter 5 are great for developing overall reactionary skills. The containment drill (page 108) adds an even greater level of sport specificity, since players must react based on the movements of the other athletes.

LACROSSE

Mike Sanders

One of the fundamental needs of most sports is locomotive agility, and this is true in the game of lacrosse.[4] In order to compete at a high level, lacrosse athletes must be able to accelerate and decelerate at high velocities while incorporating many different movement skills (side shuffling, backpedaling, cutting, drop stepping). They must also be able to perform these movements with good body control.[10, 21]

Most coaches and motor-learning experts believe that athletes can improve at a sport skill by practicing.[10] For the sake of simplicity, this section will not discuss the exact physiological theory behind skill improvement and acquisition. However, one point that can provide a better understanding of agility and quickness training is that during physical activity, muscles and joints provide proprioceptive feedback.[4, 5] As athletes repeat specific movements over and over again, the proprioceptors (i.e., muscle spindles, Golgi tendon organs) send input to the central nervous system to make it more efficient. This advancement increases the speed of muscle stimulation. In theory, these developments should improve athletes' coordination when accelerating, decelerating, and changing direction during multidirectional tasks.

An effective strength and conditioning program for lacrosse athletes should always include a planned, systematic approach to training. Agility should be part of the overall periodized plan. The goal of a well-periodized program is to systematically increase exercise stress in combination with periods of recovery in order to bring about a supercompensation response in the athlete. This means that the application of an appropriately prescribed stress to the body creates a positive adaptation.

As with any type of training, coaches should use a systematic progression for agility training. How they approach the progression depends largely on which periodized model they use. Coaches must use sound training progressions that advance athletes responsibly and safely. A strength and conditioning professional can achieve a progressive approach to agility for lacrosse in many ways. The following sections provide examples and brief explanations of agility progressions for lacrosse.

MOVEMENT DRILLS

Strength and conditioning professionals must take the necessary steps and time to touch on the basic movement patterns and postures essential to athletes' locomotion patterns. They should pay attention to foot position, leg action, posture, and arm action. For example, where should athletes place their feet during a side-shuffling drill? The coach may teach athletes how to break down their hips during deceleration to lower the center of gravity or may teach proper body posture during the acceleration phase. The preceding are only a few examples of the many body mechanic issues that coaches should address early on in the macrocycle plan. Athletes should also work through each stance and posture in a slow, controlled manner to further develop the motor patterns needed to execute each movement.

CLOSED AGILITY DRILLS

Once athletes show mastery over the basic locomotor patterns and postures, the coach should introduce closed agility drills, which have a set movement pattern and occur in a predictable and unchanging environment.[5] The *T* drill (page 85), featured in chapter 4, is an example of a closed agility drill, since athletes can anticipate the movement pattern.

OPEN AGILITY DRILLS

The next progression for athletes is to move from closed agility drills to open agility drills, which require them to accurately anticipate, read, and respond to various environmental stimuli.[5] Instead of using predetermined distances for cones that athletes can predict, the coach can use auditory cues, such as whistles or verbal commands, to indicate change of direction. Athletes can perform the same drills while responding to visual cues from the coach, such as pointing the direction, raising hands, and so on. For instance, a two-cone agility drill could progress as follows:

1. The coach removes the cones from the drill.
2. The athlete responds to the cue by sprinting forward.
3. The athlete continues to sprint until cued to change direction and side shuffle.
4. The athlete continues to side shuffle until cued to change direction and shuffle in the opposite direction.
5. The athlete continues in this direction until cued to stop and shuffle in the original direction.
6. The athlete continues to side shuffle until cued to change direction and backpedal.
7. The athlete continues to backpedal until cued to stop.

Another way to incorporate cues is to position athletes across from one another in a shadowing drill, as discussed in chapter 5 (page 105). For instance, a two-cone agility drill could progress in the following manner:

1. The coach removes the cones from the drill.
2. Athletes stand facing each other 10 to 20 yards (9–18 m) apart.
3. One athlete is assigned as the leader and the other is the follower.
4. The leader sprints forward. The follower reacts by sprinting backward.
5. The leader changes to a side shuffle and the follower reacts by side shuffling in the same direction.
6. The leader changes direction and side shuffles in the opposite direction. The follower reacts and shadows the leader.
7. The leader changes direction and side shuffles back in the original direction. The follower reacts and shadows the leader.
8. The leader changes direction again and switches to a backpedal. The follower reacts, and both athletes move through the finish.

SPORT SPECIFICITY AND ENERGY-SYSTEM STRESS

Coaches can incorporate implements, such as lacrosse sticks and balls, to make drills more specific to the sport. For example, players can hold the stick and move the ball as they go through the agility drills. The coach can further the development and difficulty of drills by adding energy-system stress. Coaches should only use this next progression when athletes demonstrate mastery and skill over the existing drills and steps. Coaches add energy-system stress by incorporating work-rest ratios into the agility program. Athletes must maintain proper footwork and posture while being timed. This, of course, adds a high level of difficulty to the drill. More difficulty can be added to the drill by including previously mentioned aspects, such as adding cues, mirroring, and using implements.

SOCCER

Ian Jeffreys

Soccer is one of the most challenging games for the strength and conditioning professional to program since it consists of almost constant movement over two 45-minute periods. Given the amount of movement in a game, agility becomes a crucial element in the effectiveness of a soccer player. Training that improves this capacity has the ability to significantly enhance soccer performance, contributing to improvement in all elements of play.

A key factor in developing agility is that it is very specific to context. Although fundamental movement patterns do exist, the ultimate aim of training is to enable players to deploy these movements effectively in a game. To this end, it is useful to think of agility as game speed (not to be confused with linear speed). *Game speed* can be defined as a context-specific skill, in which athletes maximize their performance by applying sport-specific movements of optimal velocity, precision, efficiency, and control in anticipation of and in response to the key perceptual stimuli and skill requirements of the game.[11]

This definition has a number of crucial messages. The first is that movement requirements are specific to a given sport, often even to a given position. For example, a goalkeeper's movement requirements are different from those of a central midfielder. Secondly, effective game speed consists of an optimal velocity. It should be judged by maximal velocity as well as by its precision, control, and efficiency. These terms are crucial in the context of soccer, where movements need to be maintained for a 90-minute period. Here, the ultimate aim of the game is to express soccer skills, rather than to simply move at maximal speed. Although maximal speed is an important variable, the ability to harness speed and agility to maximize soccer performance is more important.

Since game speed and agility are context specific, coaches must be able to break down the movement requirements of soccer to develop an effective program. Soccer movement is intermittent, with each game featuring between 1,000 and 1,200 bouts of movement. These movements vary in speed and direction. Typical sprinting activities span approximately 5 to 15 meters (5–16 yd) and occur once every 30 seconds on average. The majority of players' time is spent in transitional phases, where speeds vary from walking to high-speed running. These transitional movements occur in many directions, including forward, sideways, and backward. Sprinting activities can be performed straight ahead. However, they often include some change of direction, either at the outset of the sprint or at some point during it.

PROGRAM DESIGN

Given the vast range of movement requirements across 90 minutes of play and the different requirements of playing positions, the ability to develop soccer-specific agility sessions may appear daunting. However, by analyzing the targeted movement specifications of the sport, coaches can classify soccer movements and put them into a basic structure for building an effective agility program.

In order to break down soccer movements, it is helpful to ascertain what athletes are trying to achieve. Coaches can effectively carry this out using target classifications. At any given time, athletes are likely attempting to either start movement or change the direction of movement (termed *initiation movements*), trying to move at maximal velocity (*actualization movements*), or waiting in transition to react to a soccer-specific stimulus (*transition movements*). Although agility training often focuses on initiation and actualization movements, far less emphasis is placed on transition movements. Often, when these are trained, they are taught incorrectly, with the emphasis on movement speed rather than on control. Athletes' ability to start and move at maximal velocity often depends on their being in the correct position to enable effective subsequent movement. Table 7.2 on page 146 identifies the following key movements within each movement classification.

Effective agility training balances the requirements of the exercise and the ability of the athlete. Thus, a session designed for an elite athlete should look different from a session for a beginner. For this reason, a soccer-specific agility program should include a progression in movement challenge and complexity as athletes move through their stages of development. In the initial stages, athletes can benefit from closed drills (i.e., drills in which the movement is preplanned and the athlete is free to concentrate solely on the movement pattern at hand). The speed of these drills can be controlled. They often consist of single movement patterns (e.g., shuffling). In this stage, coaches should develop athletes' ability in all of the identified movement patterns for soccer to ensure that no weak links in movement ability exist. The following list provides the system for game-speed development, which shows stages of movement ability and application.[11] As athletes maintain proper movement patterns at one stage, they can progress to the next level. Athletes should do the following*:

1. Develop general and stable fundamental movement patterns.
2. Develop key movement combinations, moving from closed to open drills.
3. Develop sport-specific movements in game context.
4. Perform sport-specific movements in game context.

*© 2009 *Gamespeed: Movement Training for Superior Sports Performance* by Ian Jeffreys, Coaches Choice.

Table 7.2 Movement Patterns in Soccer

Movement type	Aim	Movement pattern
Initiation	Start to the front	Acceleration pattern
	Start to the side	Cross step
	Start to the rear	Drop step
	Change direction (linear or lateral)	Cut step or plant step
Transition	Static wait	Athletic position
	Semistatic transition: jockeying	Jockeying action
	Moving to the side	Side shuffle
	Moving to the rear	Backpedal
	Tracking the attacker diagonally	Cross-step run
	Deceleration	Deceleration pattern
	Controlled movement to the front	Chop steps in athletic position or adjustment steps
Actualization	Acceleration	Acceleration movement patterns
	Move to top speed	Kick from a rolling start, maximum speed pattern

© 2009 *Gamespeed: Movement Training for Superior Sports Performance* by Ian Jeffreys, Coaches Choice.

As athletes develop, their coaches should start to combine their movement patterns in ways typical to soccer. For example, backpedal drills can conclude with sprints to the rear, to the side, or forward. These combinations are commonly seen in soccer. As athletes develop, coaches can also deploy drills that are increasingly open. Here, athletes should respond to a range of stimuli, which can become increasingly soccer specific. For example, athletes can initiate incorporating backpedaling into a sprint drill. Next, they can change direction in response to a coach's signal, and then in response to another athlete's movement. In this way, the movement patterns become increasingly challenging in a way that progressively reflects the specific movement patterns found in soccer. These types of drills can include great variety in terms of distances, speeds, directions, and stimuli.

QUALITY IS VITAL

Practice makes permanent. This is a crucial message for any soccer agility program. If athletes are to develop effective agility, then they must perform each drill with the appropriate technique. They must always remember that the drill is merely a means to an end, and that end is enhanced agility. If they perform the drill poorly, they will not develop optimal agility. Therefore, coaches should always emphasize technique during exercises.

The movements outlined in table 7.2 provide an ideal reference for athletes to assess their performance of each movement. The results can form the start of an agility development program. Where deficiencies are seen, athletes can do additional work to bring these movements up to standard. From there, coaches can develop each movement pattern along the following continuum, which moves from basic, closed drills to random sport-specific movements that display high levels of agility. With this structure, coaches can develop soccer-specific agility for each movement pattern in table 7.2 in the following manner:

1. Develop individual movement patterns.
2. Add variation (distance and direction).
3. Develop movement combinations.
4. Move to increasingly open situations.
5. Add sport-specific requirements.

Coaches can then structure agility-development programs to ensure that all movement patterns are developed within a given time frame. This may be weekly or biweekly.

Table 7.3 on page 148 outlines a sample weekly structure that incorporates agility and speed work into warm-up protocols. This combination is a very time-efficient way of deploying a good deal of speed and agility training. It also ensures that athletes can carry out agility work when they are not fatigued.

Table 7.3 Sample Program Week Using Four Warm-Ups

Session number	Agility and speed-work focus	Drills and exercises
1	Starting and acceleration	• Starting mechanics (all directions) • Acceleration (varied directions, distances, static and rolling starts)
2	Deceleration and transition	• Mechanics of deceleration and jockeying • Jockeying and transition challenges • Challenges with applied offensive and defensive movement
3	Maximum speed	• Speed mechanics • Speed application (straight and curved runs) • Applied speed challenges
4	Direction change and applied agility	• Direction change development drills • Applied offensive and defensive movement challenges

SAMPLE AGILITY AND QUICKNESS SESSION

The following is a sample session for developing change-of-direction speed and quickness. Athletes should begin with a dynamic warm-up to prepare the body for more vigorous activity. Chapter 4 provides a variety of dynamic warm-up drills (see page 56–61) to choose from.

Lateral Shuffle and Stick

Two cones are placed 5 to 10 yards (5–9 m) apart. The athlete begins in an athletic position facing cone 1. When ready, she shuffles to cone 2 while keeping the hips low and the hips, shoulders, and torso parallel to the cones. When the athlete reaches it, she immediately sticks the finish position. The feet should be almost flat, pointed forward, and wider apart than the knees. In turn, the knees should be wider than the hips. The athlete holds the position for a brief pause to make sure she can maintain it in a stable manner. No additional movements should occur during the pause. Once stability is achieved, another movement can be started.

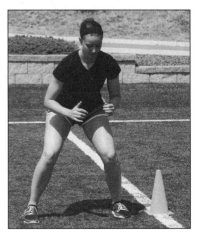

Proper finish position.

Lateral Shuffle and Push Back

Two cones are placed 5 to 10 yards (5–9 m) apart. The athlete begins in an athletic position facing cone 1. He moves laterally from cone 1 to cone 2. When he reaches it, the athlete plants the outside leg and explosively pushes back to move in the opposite direction.

Lateral Shuffle Mirror

Two cones are placed 10 yards (9 m) apart. Between the cones, two athletes assume an athletic position facing each other. One assumes the role of the offense and the other of the defense. Moving only laterally between the cones, the offensive athlete tries to lose the defensive athlete, who in turn tries to stay with the offensive athlete. The drill should last between three and six seconds.

Run to Cone and Cut

Two cones are placed 5 yards (5 m) apart. The athlete assumes an athletic position next to cone 1 and faces cone 2. With a self-start, the athlete runs toward cone 2. When she reaches it, she makes a cut step and then accelerates in the opposite direction

Coach's Signal Variation

For an open version of this drill (see photo), the coach stands 2 yards (2 m) behind cone 2. The athlete runs toward cone 2 as before, but before she reaches it, the coach gives a verbal or a visual signal instructing the athlete to move in a certain direction. The athlete makes a cut step and accelerates in the given direction.

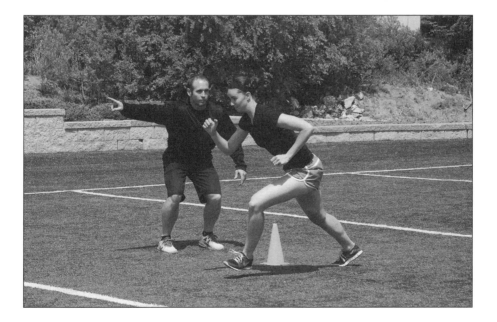

Run and Cut

For this drill (also known as get pasts), two cones are placed 10 yards (9 m) apart. Two athletes perform the drill: One assumes an offensive role and the other assumes a defensive role. The offensive athlete starts at cone 1. The defensive athlete assumes an athletic position at cone 2. The drill starts with the first movement of the offensive athlete, who moves forward trying to get to the end of the zone (cone 2). The defensive athlete moves forward and then adjusts his movements as he tries to tag the offensive athlete. The depth of the zone can be adjusted as needed based on how long the drill lasts, the skill level of the athletes, or the intended outcome of the drill. The zone can be expanded to 15 yards or even 20 yards (14–18 m), 5 or 10 yards (5–9 m) past cone 2.

Get to the Point

Two goals (or two pairs of cones) are placed 10 yards (9 m) apart. This drill is similar to the run and cut, but this time, the defender starts a few feet away from the offensive player, as in a game situation. On the coach's signal, the offensive player tries to cut and move to either the near post or the far post. To add another element of realism, another player can deliver a ball to the offensive player on the cut toward the goal. The attacker tries to direct the ball into the goal and the defender tries to clear it (as in a game).

TENNIS

Mark Kovacs

Tennis is a sport that has changed substantially over the last two decades as technology has developed and training has improved. The players who are the most successful are also the best all-around athletes. Agility and quickness are two of the most important physical components of success on the court. Training for tennis-specific quickness and agility is framed within the dimensions of movement, time, and distance covered during points. Tennis movement is highly situation specific, and it is performed in a reactive environment.[16] Although all players have some consistent traits, tennis movement is highly specific to the position of the athlete on the court and the type of shot that has just been made by the opponent.

In competitive tennis, the average point is made in less than 10 seconds.[14, 15] The recovery between points is usually between 20 and 25 seconds. Tennis players make an average of four directional changes per point,[17, 26] but motion in any given point can range from a single movement to more than 15 directional changes during a long rally. In a competitive match, it is not uncommon for players to make more than 1,000 directional changes.

Approximately 80 percent of all strokes are played within a distance less than 8 yards (7 m). Less than 5 percent of strokes are played that require more than 15 feet (5 m) between strokes.[7] It is interesting to note that tennis players can cover about 1 to 2 feet (30–60 cm) more on their forehand side than on their backhand side.[32] This piece of information is very helpful when devising movement-training programs for tennis, since athletes may need to train for slightly longer distances on the forehand side. These are important findings, since most quickness and agility programs for other sports focus on distances longer than those seen in tennis. Tennis players rarely achieve distances in which a traditional full-acceleration technique is reached. They never experience maximum velocity while running during the confines of a match.

Unlike many other sports, the majority of tennis movements are in a lateral direction. A study of professional players' movement found that more than 70 percent of movements were made from side to side, with less than 20 percent of movements in a forward, linear direction and less than 8 percent of movements in a backward, linear direction.[32] This is a vitally important statistic because lateral acceleration and deceleration in the distances previously described are the major determining factors in great tennis movement. Linear acceleration, linear maximum velocity, and agility are all separate and distinct biomotor skills that need to be trained separately[33] since training one biomotor skill does not directly affect the improvement of the other. Therefore, tennis players should focus between 60 and 80 percent of training time on lateral movements, 10 to 30 percent on linear forward movements, and only about 10 percent on linear backward movement.

One other area that can have an immediate effect on how fast athletes move in short distances is their reaction time. *Reaction time* is defined as the time between when a stimulus is detected (visual awareness of the opponent's stroke or ball) and force is produced.[28] Although reaction time does not correlate well with sprints that last longer than a few seconds, it does correlate very well with distances typically seen in tennis play.[22] Therefore, tennis athletes should train to improve reaction time along with other tennis movements, such as technique, strength, and power. In the training drills, coaches should use a visual stimulus to help athletes develop visual reaction time. An auditory stimulus (whistle, voice, or hand clap) is less tennis specific than a visual cue.

Rotation is a major component of tennis-specific movement. Movements that incorporate this skill must be used in quickness and agility drills. Many of the drills outlined in chapters 4 and 5 can be made more tennis specific by adding rotation (through the use of medicine balls or tennis strokes) during many of the change-of-direction movements. An example is to perform the drills using a tennis racket. During each change of direction, the athlete can mimic a forehand or backhand groundstroke, or even a volley. Some particularly useful drills from chapter 4 include lateral line hops and the 180-degree traveling line hop from the line drills section as well as lateral shuffle, pro-agility drill, *T* drill, and attack and retreat drill from the cone drills sections.

The following tips can be helpful when training for tennis-specific agility and quickness:

▶ Reactive drills are the goal of a tennis-specific quickness and agility program.

▶ Lateral training needs to make up the largest percentage of training time.

▶ Short distances that mimic the movement demands lead to an effective program.

▶ Coaches should track each player's movement patterns during competition and devise an individual program based on their observations.

▶ Athletes should only add resistance to exercises once they have perfected technique and movement mechanics and maintained or increased power output.

▶ Deceleration training is important to help tennis athletes move more efficiently on the court, as well as to reduce the likelihood of injury.

VOLLEYBALL

Michael Doscher

Volleyball requires multidirectional movements and jumping. A typical match is built around short, explosive bursts of movement and relatively long rest periods that allow athletes to fully recover. Rallies in volleyball generally last between 3 and 45 seconds. Depending on their position, athletes are rarely required to move more than 5 to 15 feet (1.5–5 m) in any direction. In volleyball, reacting quickly and explosively in a lateral, linear, and vertical manner is very important for optimal performance. With this in mind, coaches must develop a program that will enhance players' ability to react and move in these directions.

Reaction in any sport is the beginning of quickness. Athletes must learn how to recognize and interpret what is happening around them, and then react properly to the stimuli so they can perform the correct skill needed for the game situation. Thus, for volleyball athletes, working on first-step quickness is vital because speed is required to react quickly to a rapidly moving or spiked ball coming over the net.

DRILL SELECTION

Any of the drills listed in this book are beneficial for improving athleticism. The drills in this section were chosen based on their similarity to movements that occur in competition. Coaches should initially emphasize simple drills. As athletes master them, coaches can increase the difficulty of the drill or select more challenging drills. When applicable, athletes should perform all drills in both directions, using two-leg and single-leg variations, to challenge their balance and to increase variety and difficulty. Athletes can perform drills on a volleyball court, grass, or sand, either indoors or outdoors, to add different stimuli to the training program.

Change-of-direction drills help athletes move fluently and quickly on the court. The drills in this section help with change of direction. Any of the line, ladder, or dot drills featured in chapter 4 are excellent for improving these skills. Additionally, cone drills that cover the same approximate distances required of athletes on the court, such as most of the two-cone drills in chapter 4, are great for developing technique mastery.

Coaches should begin with drills that focus on change of direction, and then eventually progress to drills that require reaction, timing of movement, first-step quickness, and starting acceleration. These drills should not be used as methods of conditioning. Work-to-rest ratios of quickness drills should mirror those of a match. Coaches should allow athletes even more rest than they would experience in a game setting to promote recovery and maximal effort. However, occasionally, coaches can integrate drills into various parts of a workout session to help athletes perform in different states of fatigue. This practice simulates a game experience during training. However, athletes should not be so fatigued that they cannot maintain proper form and technique.

Coaches can use a variety of drills to develop the aforementioned attributes. The jump, squat, and push-up drill (page 99), quickness box drill (page 100), and Y drill (page 101) from chapter 5 are useful. The Y drill can be progressed to use different movement patterns. Coaches can also use the following drills, which include some variations on existing drills from chapters 4 and 5, as well as two new drills.

Ball Drops Drill

This drill is performed as discussed in chapter 5 on page 97. A coach or partner can vary the basic drill by holding tennis balls in each hand and dropping one to the side. The athlete doesn't know which side. The distance between athlete and coach or partner can be determined by the distance the athlete can cover. The athlete can perform the drill by moving laterally, turning, and opening on command to find the ball or by moving diagonally at different angles. Another variation is to have a coach or partner toss the balls in different directions. The athlete reacts to the ball's movement and runs to catch it before the second bounce.

Shadow Drill

This drill is performed as discussed in chapter 5 on page 105. Instead of facing each other between two cones, two athletes can set themselves up on one half of the volleyball court. The partner who is leading should perform forward runs, backward runs, lateral movements, and diagonal movements. The athletes need plenty of space between them so that the players do not run into each other on forward runs.

Shuffle Reaction Ball Drill

This drill is performed in the same manner discussed in chapter 5 on page 96. Instead of tossing a ball to the athlete, the coach or partner rolls volleyballs on the ground to the cones on the left and right of the athlete. This forces the player to stay in a low position while moving laterally. The coach or partner can vary when he releases the ball to change up the movement pattern and reaction time. The athlete will go for a set period of time.

Four-Cone Reaction Box

Four cones are placed in a square pattern. The size of box will be determined by how much movement is desired, the position of the athlete, and what is desired from the drill. The player starts in the center of the box. A partner or coach gives directional cues for the athlete to react to. The athlete runs to different cones for a set period of time or a set number of repetitions.

Six-Cone Quickness Drill

Six cones are set up in a hexagon pattern. Coaches can determine the size of the pattern by the athlete's size, stride, or limb length. From the center of the pattern, the athlete should be able to reach each cone on one stride. The coach gives the athlete cues about which cone to step to. The cues can be visual, such as pointing to a specific cone, or auditory in which case the cones need to be different colors or numbered. The athlete should make contact with the named cone and then return back to the center to wait for another directional cue. The drill is finished when the athlete has touched all the cones or a predetermined amount of time is complete. This drill can be performed with the athlete facing one direction throughout the drill or with the athlete opening the hips and moving in multiple movement patterns.

Sport-specific drills are the last key to volleyball agility training. Athletes can accomplish them by performing dry runs of offensive plays and defense plays without the ball. Coaches should make sure that athletes move in the right manner and with the proper technique.

PROGRAM DESIGN

The foundation to training is to add variety to the drills every three to four weeks, or once athletes have mastered a drill. The overall goal is to make athletes less prone to injuries and more athletic. Designing a training program begins with dividing the year into different parts, based on the type of training needed and the amount of competition occurring. The following sections provide guidelines for each part. Coaches should modify them based on athletes' level and ability.

Postseason (2 to 4 Weeks)

The time after the season should be for active recovery. During this phase, athletes should ideally perform two sets of two or three lower-intensity drills once a week. Athletes should work on technique, so that when they start doing drills at full speed, they will move quickly and fluently. They should use the majority of this time for active recovery and cross-training.

Off-Season (6 to 12 Weeks)

During this time, drill volumes should start to get higher. Athletes can train two times a week for speed, agility and quickness, and power. Athletes should select drills that vary in difficulty from low to moderate, and should perform four to six drills, with three or four reps per drill. Plyometric drills, such as dot drills (see page 75), can be added at this time. Athletes should begin by performing two to four exercises of low to moderate intensity for no more than 120 contacts per session.

Preseason (6 to 12 Weeks)

During this time, drill volumes are at their highest in the beginning, but then taper to moderate by the end. Athletes should perform drills three times a week, doing six to eight drills and four to six reps of each drill. They should start to increase the intensity of plyometric drills from moderate to high, performing five to eight drills, with a total of 250 contacts.

In-Season (3 to 5 Months)

During this time, the athletes' drills should be purely sport specific. They may use other drills to warm up. They should perform a low volume of one or two drills for one or two reps. Any plyometrics that athletes use at this time should be low-level warm-ups, since they will be doing a lot of jumping in practice and games.

WRESTLING

Greg Infantolino

Many factors are involved in the development of an elite wrestler. Along with skill, ability, and mastery of technique, wrestlers must possess high levels of dynamic and isometric strength, anaerobic conditioning, balance, quickness, power, and agility.[13] Wrestlers don't need to cover large distances; they just have to be able to cover the mat as quickly as possible. Therefore, the strength and conditioning professional must develop a program that will improve wrestlers' production of force and increase their agility and quickness in order to improve their ability to execute the fast movements needed to respond to an opponent's attack or to explode offensively.

Wrestlers must be quick and powerful in an attempt to take down, throw, turn, or defend an opponent's attack. They must also have the endurance to compete for an entire match.[29] Wrestling is primarily an anaerobic sport that taxes both the ATP-CP and lactic-acid energy systems.[18] Approximately 90 percent of the energy needed to complete a wrestling match is derived from the phosphagen and lactic-acid energy systems.[12] Therefore, wrestlers must be able to buffer high amounts of lactic-acid buildup in order to maintain optimal strength and power during competition.[19] Thus, coaches must use the appropriate type of training program to develop the physiological adaptations that wrestlers need to be quick and explosive over a five-minute period.

Anaerobic sports, such as wrestling, demand high levels of force during movements. Sometimes, athletes must perform in a fatigued state. As a result, wrestlers need to condition their fast-twitch muscle fibers and their capacity to perform extended periods of work.[12] Since wrestling is a high-intensity sport, in which matches are usually won or lost in a flurry of explosive offensive and defensive maneuvers, interval agility training is highly applicable to the sport's conditioning needs.[19] Agility is a trainable motor skill that any athlete can improve through proper repetition.

NEUROMUSCULAR TRAINING

Agility and quickness training falls under the category of neuromuscular training. Neuromuscular training creates better body awareness, balance, and coordination, in order to increase reaction time and effectiveness.[1] No matter an athlete's skill level, he is at a major disadvantage if he is slower than his opponent. General agility, quickness, and movement training improves body awareness, balance, and change-of-direction speed.[27]

Wrestlers must train to move in every direction so they can explode to the front, to the back, and laterally. Enhancing agility will help them defend or attack at any moment. The strength and conditioning professional can have some flexibility in developing the agility program by adjusting the duration of the agility drill, the rest intervals, the repetitions, or the number of sets performed, depending on the time of year and the desired training effect.

PROGRAM DESIGN

For agility and quickness training, athletes should work on three or four different drills that emphasize change-of-direction speed. These drills should be performed in rotation anywhere from one to four days a week, depending on the competitive season. Athletes should cycle through a variety of drills to keep the training fresh and to move the body in multiple directions. Coaches can program these drills with a set pattern or as reaction drills, in which wrestlers respond to a visual cue. The athletes' focus during these drills should be on the quality of repetitions, not the quantity. Coaches should terminate the drill when the athletes' exercise technique is compromised due to fatigue.

Many of the agility and quickness drills from chapters 4 and 5 can be used in wrestling training programs. The following drills and variations for those drills are useful for wrestlers:

▶ *Pro-agility drill* (page 82). The athlete completes the basic drill once by sprinting. Then, he does the drill a second time using carioca and a third time using shuffling. Changing how the athlete moves through this drill mimics different movement patterns that wrestlers need. In most cases, wrestlers do not move in specifically linear or lateral patterns. However, by adding a variety of specific movements that are performed during a match, the athlete may improve agility and quickness.

▶ *Four-cone drills.* This includes the X drill (page 88) and the four corners drill (page 86). For the four corners drill, the athlete should use the following movement patterns:
  • Sprint, backpedal, shuffle, sprint
  • Sprint, carioca, backpedal, shuffle

▶ *Five-cone drills* (page 89–92). This includes the attack and retreat, M, and hourglass drills.

▶ *Reactive drills.* This includes the quickness box (page 100), shadow drill (page 105), knee tag (page 110), and jump, squat, push-up (page 99).

▶ *Line drills* (page 61–64). When completing these drills, the athlete should spend as little time on the ground as possible with each hop. He should cover the distance over the line as quickly as possible. Doing so helps the wrestler explode with quickness and balance, enabling him to quickly cover a short distance in a match. Wrestlers who can control balance and coordination can more efficiently perform wrestling moves immediately after an explosive movement.

Agility Shuttle

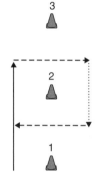

This drill is great for developing explosiveness, foot speed, balance, quickness, and agility, which are all needed during a match. It also improves the ability to accelerate, decelerate, and perform movements in all directions. Ten cones are set up in a straight line with 3 feet (1 m) between the cones. The athlete begins in an athletic position to the left side of cone 1. The athlete sprints to a point just past cone 2, then breaks down and shuffles to the right just past cone 2, backpedals to just behind cone 2, and then shuffles back to the left of cone 2 (see illustration). From there, the athlete sprints to cone 3 and then repeats the same pattern at this cone and at each of the remaining cones in the line. After completing this run, the athlete should rest one minute between attempts. Then, the athlete repeats the drill, beginning this time to the right of cone 1. During the drill, the athlete's hips must stay low during each change of direction. He should maintain balance and body control at all times. The body should not lean backward during the backpedaling or too far to the side during the shuffling.

Get-Ups

In most matches, wrestlers find themselves on the mat on their back, side, or abdomen. The ability to recover quickly and to move into a position to come back at an opponent is key to success for wrestlers. This drill helps wrestlers develop quickness and agility while improving their ability to recover from being put on their backs or thrown to the mat. Between 15 and 20 cones are set up around the wrestling mat to form a square. The cones should be numbered. The cones should be 3 to 8 yards (3–7 m) away from the center of the mat. The athlete lies down in the center with the back on the mat. The coach gives a *go* command followed by a cone number. On the *go* command, the athlete rolls over, gets to his feet as quickly as possible, and sprints to the designated cone. The athlete comes back to the center of the mat, lies down again, and repeats the drill, running to a different cone each time. He repeats the drill for four to six reps, with a 45-second rest between runs. The athlete must maintain body control and balance when rolling over to get up from the mat. He should eliminate wasted motion to improve how quickly he can get up and recover from being on the mat. For variety, the cone pattern can be varied.

References

Introduction

1. Abernethy, B. (1999). Anticipation in squash: Differences in advance cue utilization between expert and novice. *Journal of Sports Sciences, 8,* 17-34.

2. Abernethy, B., & Russell, D.G. (1987). Expert-novice difference in an applied selective attention task. *Journal of Sport Psychology, 9,* 326-345.

3. Baker, D., & Nance, S. (1999). The relationship between running speed and measures of strength and power in professional rugby league players. *Journal of Strength and Conditioning Research, 13,* 230-235.

4. Djevalikian, R. (1993). *The relationship between asymmetrical leg power and change of running direction.* Chapel Hill: University of North Carolina.

5. Farrow, D., & Abernethy, B. (2002). Can anticipatory skills be learned through implicit video-based perceptual training? *Journal of Sports Sciences, 20,* 471-485.

6. Webb, P., & Lander, J. (1983). An economical fitness testing battery for high school and college rugby teams. *Sports Coach, 7,* 44-46.

7. Young, W.B., James, R., & Montgomery, I. (2002). Is muscle power related to running speed with changes of direction? *Journal of Sports Medicine and Physical Fitness, 43,* 282-288.

Chapter 1

1. Aagaard, P., Simonsen, E.B., Andersen, J.L., Magnusson, P., & Dyhre-Poulsen, P. (2002). Increased rate of force development and neural drive of human skeletal muscle following resistance training. *J Appl Physiol, 93*(4), 1318-1326.

2. Baker, D., Wilson, G., & Carlyon, R. (1994). Periodization: The effect on strength of manipulating volume and intensity. *J Strength Cond Res, 8*(4), 235-42.

3. Bale, P., Mayhew, J.L., Piper, F.C., Ball, T.E., & Willman, M.K. (1992). Biological and performance variables in relation to age in male and female adolescent athletes. *J Sports Med Phys Fitness, 32*(2), 142-148.

4. Blackburn, J.T., Mynark, R.G., Padua, D.A., & Guskiewicz, K.M. (2006). Influences of experimental factors on spinal stretch reflex latency and amplitude in the human triceps surae. *J Electromyogr Kinesiol, 16*(1),42-50.

5. Bosco, C., Komi, P.V., & Ito, A. (1981). Prestretch potentiation of human skeletal muscle during ballistic movement. *Acta Physiol Scand, 111*(2), 135-140.

6. Brindle, T.J., Nyland, J., Shapiro, R., Caborn, D.N., & Stine, R. (1999). Shoulder proprioception: latent muscle reaction times. *Med Sci Sports Exerc, 31*(10), 1394-1398.

7. Callan, S.D., Brunner, D.M., Devolve, K.L., Mulligan, S.E., Hesson, J., Wilber, R.L., & Kennedy, J.T. (2000) Physiological profiles of elite freestyle wrestlers. *Journal of Strength and Conditioning Research, 14*(2), 162-169.

8. Carlock, J.M., Smith, S.L., Hartman, M.J., Morris, R.T., Ciroslan, D.A., Pierce, K.C., et al. (2004). The relationship between vertical jump power estimates and weightlifting ability: A field-test approach. *J Strength Cond Res, 18*(3), 534-539.

9. Chappell, J.D., & Limpisvasti, O. (2008). Effect of a neuromuscular training program on the kinetics and kinematics of jumping tasks. *Am J Sports Med, 36*(6), 1081-1086.

10. Cissik, J.M. (2004). Means and methods of speed training, part I. *Strength and Conditioning Journal, 26*(4), 24-29.

11. Cissik, J.M., & Barnes, M. (2004). *Sport speed and agility.* Monterey CA: Coaches Choice.

12. Claessens, A.L., Lefevre, J., Beunen, G., & Malina, R.M. (1999) The contribution of anthropometric characteristics to performance scores in elite female gymnasts. *Journal of Sports Medicine and Physical Fitness, 39*(4), 355-360.

13. Deane, R.S., Chow, J.W., Tillman, M.D., & Fournier, K.A. (2005). Effects of hip flexor training on sprint, shuttle run, and vertical jump performance. *J Strength Cond Res, 19*(3), 615-621.

14. Enoka, R. (2002). *Neuromechanics of human movement* (3rd ed.). Champaign, IL: Human Kinetics.

15. Flynn, T.W., & Soutas-Little, R.W. (1993). Mechanical power and muscle action during forward and backward running. *J Orthop Sports Phys Ther, 17*(2), 108-112.

16. Garrett, W.E., Jr. (1990). Muscle strain injuries: Clinical and basic aspects. *Med Sci Sports Exerc, 22*(4), 436-443.

17. Goodman, C. (2009). Improving agility techniques. *NSCA's Performance Training Journal, 7*(4), 10-12.

18. Hakkinen, K., Komi, P.V., & Alen, M. (1985). Effect of explosive type strength training on isometric force- and relaxation-time, electromyographic and muscle fibre characteristics of leg extensor muscles. *Acta Physiol Scand, 125*(4), 587-600.

19. Ham, D.J., Knez, W.L., & Young, W.B. (2007). A deterministic model of the vertical jump: Implications for training. *J Strength Cond Res, 21*(3), 967-972.

20. Harland, M.J., & Steele, J.R. 1997. Biomechanics of the sprint start. *Sports Med 1997, 23*(1), 11-20.

21. Harman, E. (2008). Biomechanics of resistance exercise. In T.R. Baechle & R.W. Earle, (Eds.). *Essentials of strength training and conditioning* (3rd ed., pp. 66-91). Champaign, IL: Human Kinetics.

22. Haywood, K.M., & Getchell, N. (2005). *Life span motor development* (4th ed.). Champaign, IL: Human Kinetics.

23. Hefzy, M.S., al Khazim, M., & Harrison, L. (1997). Co-activation of the hamstrings and quadriceps during the lunge exercise. *Biomed Sci Instrum, 33,* 360-365.

24. Houck, J. (2003). Muscle activation patterns of selected lower extremity muscles during stepping and cutting tasks. *J Electromyogr Kinesiol, 13*(6), 545-554.

25. Kawamori, N., Rossi, S.J., Justice, B.D., Haff, E.E., Pistilli, E.E., O'Bryant, H.S., et al. (2006). Peak force and rate of force development during isometric and dynamic mid-thigh clean pulls performed at various intensities. *J Strength Cond Res, 20*(3), 483-491.

26. Khosla, T. (1984) Physique of female swimmers and divers from the 1976 Montreal Olympics. *Journal of American Medical Association, 252*(4), 536-537.

27. Knuttgen, H.G., & Kraemer, W.J. (1987). Terminology and measurement in exercise performance. *Journal of Applied Sport Science Research, 1,* 1-10.

28. Koch, A.J., O'Bryant, H.S., Stone, M.E., Sanborn, K., Proulx, C., Hruby, J., et al. (2003). Effect of warm-up on the standing broad jump in trained and untrained men and women. *J Strength Cond Res, 17*(4), 710-714.

29. Komi, P.V. (1984). Physiological and biomechanical correlates of muscle function: Effects of muscle structure and stretch-shortening cycle on force and speed. *Exerc Sport Sci Rev, 12,* 81-122.

30. Komi, P.V., & Viitasalo, J.H. (1976). Signal characteristics of EMG at different levels of muscle tension. *Acta Physiol Scand, 96*(2), 267-276.

31. Landry, S.C., McKean, K.A., Hubley-Kozey, C.L., Stanish, W.D., & Deluzio, K.J. (2007). Neuromuscular and lower limb biomechanical differences exist between male and female elite adolescent soccer players during an unanticipated run and crosscut maneuver. *Am J Sports Med, 35*(11), 1901-1111.

32. Lin, J.D., Liu, Y., Lin, J.C., Tsai, F.J., & Chao, C.Y. (2008). The effects of different stretch amplitudes on electromyographic activity during drop jumps. *J Strength Cond Res, 22*(1), 32-39.

33. Lockie, R.G., Murphy, A.J., & Spinks, C.D. (2003). Effects of resisted sled towing on sprint kinematics in field-sport athletes. *J Strength Cond Res, 17*(4), 760-767.

34. Luhtanen, P., & Komi, P.V. (1978). Mechanical factors influencing running speed. In E. Asmussen & K. Jorgensen (Eds.), *Biomechanics VI-B.* Baltimore: University Park Press.

35. Mero, A., & Komi, P.V. (1986). Force-, EMG-, and elasticity-velocity relationships at submaximal, maximal and supramaximal running speeds in sprinters. *Eur J Appl Physiol Occup Physiol, 55*(5), 553-561.

36. Myer, G.D., Ford, K.R., McLean, S.G., & Hewett, T.E. (2006). The effects of plyometric versus dynamic stabilization and balance training on lower extremity biomechanics. *Am J Sports Med, 34*(3), 445-455.

37. Peterson, M.D., Alvar, B.A., & Rhea, M.R. (2006). The contribution of maximal force production to explosive movement among young collegiate athletes. *J Strength Cond Res, 20*(4), 867-873.

38. Plisk, S.S. (2008). Speed, agility, and speed-endurance development. In T.R. Baechle & R.W. Earle (Eds.), *Essentials of strength training and conditioning* (3rd ed., p 458-485). Champaign, IL: Human Kinetics.

39. Reeberg Stagnelli, L.C., Duardo, A.C., Oncken, P., Mancan, S., & da Costa, S.C. (2008). Adaptations on jump capacity in Brazilian volleyball players prior to the under-19 world championship. *J Strength Cond Res, 22*(3), 741-749.

40. Salonikidis, K., & Zafeiridis, A. (2008) The effects of plyometric, tennis-drills, and combined training on reaction, lateral and linear speed, power, and strength in novice tennis players. *Journal of Strength and Conditioning Research, 22*(1), 182-191.

41. Sheppard, J. M., Barker, M., & Gabbett, T. (2008). Training agility in elite rugby players: A case study. *Journal of Australian Strength and Conditioning, 16*(3), 15-19.

42. Sigward, S., & Powers, C.M. (2006). The influence of experience on knee mechanics during side-step cutting in females. *Clin Biomech, 21*(7), 740-747.

43. Stone, M.H., Stone, M., & Sands, B. (2007). *Principles and practice of resistance training.* Champaign, IL: Human Kinetics.

44. Tan, B., Aziz, A.R., & Chuan, T.K. (2000) Correlations between physiological parameters and performance in elite ten-pin bowlers. *Journal of Science and Medicine in Sport, 3*(2), 176-185.

45. Taskin. (2008). Evaluating sprinting ability, density of acceleration, and speed dribbling ability of professional soccer players with respect to their positions. *Journal of Strength and Conditioning Research, 22*(5), 1481–1486.

46. Toriola, A.L., Adeniran, S.A., & Ogunremi, P.T. (1987) Body composition and anthropometric characteristics of elite male basketball and volleyball players. *Journal of Sports Medicine, 27*(2), 235-238.

47. Viitasalo, J.T., & Komi, P.V. (1981). Effects of fatigue on isometric force- and relaxation-time characteristics in human muscle. *Acta Physiol Scand, 111*(1), 87-95.

48. Wallace, B.J., Kernozek, T.W., & Bothwell, E.C. (2007). Lower extremity kinematics and kinetics of Division III collegiate baseball and softball players while performing a modified pro-agility task. *J Sports Med Phys Fitness, 47*(4), 377-384.

49. Walshe, A.D., Wilson, G.J., & Ettema, G.J. (1998). Stretch-shorten cycle compared with isometric preload: Contributions to enhanced muscular performance. *J Appl Physiol, 84*(1), 97-106.

50. Watts, P.B., Martin, D.T., & Durtschi, S. (1993) Anthropometric profiles of elite male and female competitive sport rock climbers. *Journal of Sports Sciences, 11*(2), 113-117.

51. Winchester, J.B., McBride, J.M., Maher, M.A., Mikat, R.P., Allen, B.K., Kline, D.E., et al. (2008). Eight weeks of ballistic exercise improves power independently of changes in strength and muscle fiber type expression. *J Strength Cond Res, 22*(6), 1728-1734.

52. Wisloff, U., Castagna, C., Helgerud, J., Jones, R., & Hoff, J. (2004). Strong correlation of maximal squat strength with sprint performance and vertical jump height in elite soccer players. *Br J Sports Med, 38*(3), 285-288.

53. Young, W.B., James, R., & Montgomery, I. (2002). Is muscle power related to running speed with changes of direction? *J. Sports Med. Phys. Fitness, 42,* 282-288.

54. Young, W., Wilson, G., & Byrne, C. (1999). Relationship between strength qualities and performance in standing and run-up vertical jumps. *J Sports Med Phys Fitness, 39*(4), 285-293.

55. Yu, B., Queen, R.M., Abbey, A.N., Liu, Y., Moorman, C.T., & Garrett, W.E. (2008). Hamstring muscle kinematics and activation during overground sprinting. *J Biomech, 41*(15), 3121-3126.

56. Zatsiorsky, V.M. (2003). Biomechanics of strength and strength testing. In P.V. Komi (Ed.), *Strength and power in sport* (pp. 439-487). Oxford, England: Blackwell Scientific.

Chapter 2

1. Abernethy, B., & Russell, D.G. (1987). Expert-novice difference in an applied selective attention task. *Journal of Sport Psychology, 9,* 326-345.

2. Abernethy, B., Wann, J., & Parks, S. (1998). Training perceptual-motor skills for sport. In B.C. Elliot (Ed.), *Training in Sport: Applying Sport Science* (pp. 426). West Sussex, England: Wiley.

3. Abernethy, B., Wood, M.J., & Parks, S. (1999). Can the anticipatory skills of experts be learned by novices? *Research Quarterly for Exercise and Sport, 70*(3), 331-318.

4. Baechle, T.R. & Earle, R.W. (2008). *Essentials of Strength Training and Conditioning* (3rd ed.). Champaign, IL: Human Kinetics.

5. Beashel, P., Sibson, A., & Taylor, J. (2001). *The world of sports examined* (2nd ed.). Cheltenham, England: Nelson Thornes.

6. Berry, J.T. (1999). Pattern recognition and expertise in Australian football. *School of human movement and sports sciences.* Ballarat, Australia: University of Ballarat.

7. Chelladurai, P., Yuhasz, M., & Sipura, R. (1977). The reactive agility test. *Perceptual and Motor Skills, 44,* 1319-1324.

8. Cox, R.H. (2002). *Sport psychology: Concepts and applications.* New York: McGraw-Hill.

9. Dawes, J. (2008). Creating open agility drills. *Strength and Cond. J., 30*(5), 54-55.

10. Farrow, D., & Abernethy, B. (2002). Can anticipatory skills be learned through implicit video-based perceptual training? *Journal of Sports Sciences, 20,* 471-485.

11. Farrow, D., Chivers, P., Hardingham, C., & Sachse, S. (1998). The effect of video-based perceptual training on the tennis return of serve. *International Journal of Sport Psychology, 29,* 231-242.

12. Hanin, Y.L. (2000). *Emotions in sport.* Champaign, IL: Human Kinetics.

13. Hertel, J., Denegar, C.R., Johnson, S.A., Hale, S.A., & Buckley, W.E. (1999). Reliability of the cybex reactor in the assessment of an agility task. *Journal of Sport Rehabilitation, 8,* 24-31.

14. Muir, P.A. (1996). Expertise in surfing: Nature of the perceptual advantage. Unpublished honors thesis. Ballarat, Australia: University of Ballarat.

15. Prapavesis, H., & Grove, R. (1991). Precompetitive emotions and shooting performance: The mental health and zones of optimal functioning models. *The Sport Psychologist, 5,* 223-234.

16. Ritchie, N. (1999). An investigation of pattern recognition anticipation within Australian rules football. Unpublished honors thesis. Ballarat, Australia: University of Ballarat.

17. Schmidt, R.A., & Lee, T.D. (2005). *Motor control and learning: A behavioral emphasis* (4th ed.). Champaign, IL: Human Kinetics.

18. Schmidt, R.A., & Wrisberg, C.A. (2007). *Motor learning and performance* (4th ed.). Champaign, IL: Human Kinetics.

19. Sheppard, J.M., Barker, M., & Gabbett, T. (2008). Training agility in elite rugby players: A case study. *Journal of Australian Strength and Conditioning, 16*(3), 15-19.

20. Starkes, J. (1987). Skill in field hockey: The nature of the cognitive advantage. *Journal of Sport Psychology, 9,* 146-160.

21. Tenenbaum, G., Levy-Kolker, N., Sade, S., Liebermann, D., & Lidor, R. (1996). Anticipation and confidence of decisions related to skilled performance. *International Journal of Sport Psychology, 27,* 293-307.

22. Vickers, J.N. (2007). *Perception, cognition, and decision training: The quiet eye in action.* Champaign, IL: Human Kinetics.

23. Williams, A.M., Davids, K., Burwitz, L., Williams, J.G. (1993). Visual search and sports performance. *The Australian Journal for Science and Medicine in Sport, 25*(2), 55-65.

Chapter 3

1. Hagerman, P.S. (2001). *Fitness testing 101: A guide for personal trainers and coaches.* www.iUniverse.com.

2. Harman, E. (2008). Principle of test selection and administration. In T.R. Baechle & R.W. Earle (Eds.), *Essentials of strength training and conditioning* (3rd ed., pp. 238-241). Champaign, IL: Human Kinetics.

3. Harmon, E. & Pandorf, C. (2000). Principles of test selection and administration. In T.R. Baechle & R.W. Earle (Eds.), *Essentials of strength training and conditioning* (2nd ed., pp. 276-285). Champaign, IL: Human Kinetics.

4. Klavora, P. (2000). Vertical-jump tests: A critical review. *Strength & Conditioning Journal, 22*(5), 70-75.

5. Pauoli, K., Madole, K., Garhammer, J., Lacourse, M., & Rozenek, R. (2000). Reliability and validity of the T-test as a measure of agility, leg power, and leg speed in college-aged men and women. *Journal of Strength and Conditioning Research, 14*(4), 443-450.

Chapter 4 (Works Consulted)

1. Bompa, T. (2000). *Total training for young champions.* Champaign, IL: Human Kinetics.

2. Brown, L.E., & Ferrigno, V.A. (2005). *Training for speed, agility, and quickness* (2nd ed.). Champaign, IL: Human Kinetics.

3. Cissik, J.M., & Barnes, M. (2004). *Sport speed and agility.* Monterey CA: Coaches Choice.

4. Foran, B. (2001). *High-performance sports conditioning.* Champaign, IL: Human Kinetics.

5. McHenry, P., & Raether, J. (2004). *101 agility drills.* Monterey, CA: Coaches Choice.

6. Plisk, S.S. (2000). Speed, agility, and speed-endurance development. In T.R. Baechle & R.W. Earle (Eds.), *Essentials of strength training and conditioning* (pp. 471-492). Champaign, IL: Human Kinetics.

7. Plisk, S.S. (2008). Speed, agility, and speed endurance development. In T.R. Baechle & R.W. Earle (Eds.), *Essentials of strength training and conditioning* (3rd ed., pp. 458-485). Champaign, IL: Human Kinetics.

Chapter 5 (Works Consulted)

1. Bompa, T. (2000). *Total training for young champions*. Champaign, IL: Human Kinetics.

2. Brown, L.E., & Ferrigno, V.A. (2005). *Training for speed, agility, and quickness* (2nd ed.). Champaign, IL: Human Kinetics.

3. Dawes, J. (2008) Learning to react. *Professional Strength and Conditioning*, 9: 25-27.

4. Dawes, J. (2008) One-on-one: Creating open agility drills. *Strength and Conditioning Journal*, 30(5) 54-55.

5. Dawes, J. (2009).Conditioning games for the tactical athlete, *NSCA's TSAC report, 9:* 9.4

6. Dawes, J. (2009). Reactive Six Cone Agilities, *NSCA's TSAC report,* 8: 8.9

7. Dawes, J., & Mooney, C. (2006). *101 conditioning games and drills for athletes*. Monterey, California: Monterey Bay Press.

8. Dawes, J. & Roozen, M. (2009). Reactive agility training: The shadow drill. *Tactical edge magazine.* 27(4), 82-84.

9. McHenry, P., & Raether, J. (2004). *101 agility drills*. Monterey, CA: Coaches Choice.

10. Twist, P. (2001). Lightning quickness. In B. Foran, (Ed.), *High-performance sports conditioning* (pp. 99-109). Champaign, IL: Human Kinetics.

11. Verstegen, M., & Marcello, B. (2001). Agility and coordination. In B. Foran (Ed.), *Higher performance sports conditioning* (pp.139-165). Champaign, IL: Human Kinetics.

12. Vives, D., & Roberts, J. (2005). Quickness and reaction-time training. In L.E. Brown & V.A. Ferrigno, (Eds.), *Training for speed, agility, and quickness* (2nd ed., pp. 137-195). Champaign, IL: Human Kinetics.

Chapter 6

1. Abernethy, B. (1993). Searching for the minimal essential information for skilled perception and action. *Psychol Res, 55,* 131-138.

2. Abernethy, B. (1996). Training the visual-perceptual skills of athletes. Insights from the study of motor expertise. *Am J Sports Med, 24,* S89-S92.

3. Abernethy, B., Wann, J., & Parks, S. (1998). Training perceptual motor skills for sport. In B. Elliott (Ed.), *Training for sport: Applying sport science* (pp. 1-68). Chichester, England: Wiley.

4. Abernethy, B., & Wood, J.M. (2001). Do generalized visual training programmes for sport really work? An experimental investigation. *J Sports Sci, 19,* 203-222.

5. Besier, T.F., Lloyd, D.G., Ackland, T.R., & Cochrane, J.L. (2001). Anticipatory effects on knee joint loading during running and cutting maneuvers. *Med Sci Sports Exerc, 33,* 1168-1175.

6. Besier, T.F., Lloyd, D.B., Cochrane, J.L., & Ackland, T.R. (2001). External loading of the knee joint during running and cutting maneuvers. *Med Sci Sports Exerc, 33,* 1168-1175.

7. Bompa, T. (2000). *Total training for young champions.* Champaign, IL: Human Kinetics.

8. Brittenham, G. (1996). *Complete conditioning for basketball.* Champaign, IL: Human Kinetics.

9. Cissik, J.M., & Barnes, M. (2004). *Sport speed and agility.* Monterey CA: Coaches Choice.

10. Clark, M. (2001). *Integrated training for the new millennium.* Thousand Oaks, CA: National Academy of Sports Medicine.

11. Costello, F., & Kreis, E.J. (1993). *Sports Agility.* Nashville: Taylor Sports.

12. Craig, B. (2004). What is the scientific basis of speed and agility? *NSCA Journal, 26*(3), 13-14.

13. Drabik, J. (1996). *Children & sports training: How your future champions should exercise to be healthy, fit, and happy.* Island Pond, VT: Stadion Publishing.

14. Foran, B. (2001). *High-performance sports conditioning.* Champaign, IL: Human Kinetics.

15. Fulton, K.T. (1992). Off-season strength training for basketball. *Nat Strength Cond J, 14,* 31-33.

16. Gabbert, T.J., Carius, J., & Mulvey, M. (2008). Does improved decision making ability reduce the physiological demands of game-based activities in field sport athletes? *J Str Cond Res, 22*(6), 2027-2035.

17. Gambetta, V. (1996). How to develop sport-specific speed. *Sports Coach, 19,* 22-24.

18. Kibler, W.B. (1994). Clinical biomechanics of the elbow in tennis: Implications for evaluation and diagnosis. *Med Sci Sports Exerc, 26,* 1203-1206.

19. Magill, R.A. (2006). *Motor learning and control* (8th ed.). New York: McGraw-Hill.

20. Meriam, J.L., & Kraige, L.G. (2002). *Engineering mechanics: Dynamics* (5th ed.). New York: Wiley.

21. Moreno, E. (1995). Developing quickness: Part 2. *Strength Cond, 17,* 38-39.

22. Patton, R.W., Granthan, W.C., Gerson, R.F., & Gettman, L.R. (1989). *Developing and managing health/fitness facilities.* Champaign, IL: Human Kinetics.

23. Plisk, S.S. (2000). Speed, agility, and speed-endurance development. In T.R. Baechle & R.W. Earle (Eds.), *Essentials of strength training and conditioning* (pp. 471-492). Champaign, IL: Human Kinetics.

24. Plisk, S.S. (2000). The angle on agility. *Training and Conditioning, 10*(6), 37-43.

25. Plisk, S.S. (2008). Speed, agility, and speed endurance development. In T.R. Baechle & R.W. Earle (Eds.), *Essentials of strength training and conditioning* (3rd ed., pp. 458-485). Champaign, IL: Human Kinetics.

26. Prentice, W.E., & Voight, M.I. (1999). *Techniques in musculoskeletal rehabilitation.* Chicago: McGraw-Hill.

27. Schmidt, R.A., & Lee, T.D. (2005). *Motor control and learning: A behavioral emphasis* (4th ed.). Champaign, IL: Human Kinetics.

28. Schmidt, R.A., & Wrisberg, C.A. (2007). *Motor learning and performance* (4th ed.). Champaign, IL: Human Kinetics.

29. Smythe, R. (1995). Acts of agility. *Training and Conditioning, 5.4,* August.

30. Smythe, R. (1996). Mobility + ability = agility. *Coaching Management, 4.1,* Basketball preseason.

31. Stone, M.H., Stone, M., & Sands, W.A. (2007). *Principles and practice of resistance training.* Champaign, IL: Human Kinetics.

32. Tharrett, A.J., McInnis, K.J., & Peterson, J.A. (2007). *ACSM's health/fitness facility standards and guidelines* (3rd ed.). Champaign, IL: Human Kinetics.

33. Verstegen, M., & Marcello, B. (2001). Agility and coordination. In B. Foran (Ed.), *Higher performance sports conditioning* (pp.139-165). Champaign, IL: Human Kinetics.

34. Vives, D., & Roberts, J. (2005). Quickness and reaction-time training. In L.E. Brown & V.A. Ferrigno, (Eds.), *Training for speed, agility, and quickness* (2nd ed., pp. 137-195). Champaign, IL: Human Kinetics.

35. Wathen, M.S., Baechel, T.R., & Earle, R.W. (2008). Periodization. In T.R. Baechle & R.W. Earle (Eds.), *Essentials of strength training and conditioning* (3rd ed.). Champaign, IL: Human Kinetics.

36. Wilmore, J.H., & Costill, D.L. (2004) *Physiology of sport and exercise* (3rd ed.). Champaign, IL: Human Kinetics.

Chapter 7

1. Brown, K. (2009). Speed, agility, and quickness training: No pain all gain. *NSCA Performance Journal, 8*(4): 17-18.

2. Brown, L.E., & Ferrigno, V.A. (2005). *Training for speed, agility, and quickness* (2nd ed.). Champaign, IL: Human Kinetics.

3. Cissik, J.M., & Barnes, M. (2004). *Sport speed and agility.* Monterey Bay, CA: Coaches Choice.

4. Craig, B. (2004). What is the scientific basis of speed and agility? *Strength and Cond. J., 26*(3), 13-14.

5. Dawes, J. (2008). Creating open agility drills. *Strength and Cond. J., 30*(5), 54-55.

6. Enoka, R.M. (2002). *Neuromechanics of human movement* (3rd ed.). Champaign, IL: Human Kinetics.

7. Ferrauti, A., & Weber, K. (2001). *Stroke situations in clay court tennis.* Unpublished data.

8. Gambetta, V. (2004). The right moves. *Coaching Management, 12*(4), 39-44.

9. Green, M.R., Pivarnik, J.M., Carrier, D.P., & Womack, C.J. (2006). Relationship between physiological profiles and on-ice performance of a National Collegiate Athletic Association Division I hockey team. *J Strength Cond Res, 20*(1), 43-46.

10. Jeffreys, I. (2006). Motor learning: Applications for agility, part 1. *Strength and Cond. J., 28,* 72-76.

11. Jeffreys, I. (2009). *Gamespeed: Movement training for superior sports performance.* Monterey, CA: Coaches Choice.

12. Kell, R. (1997). The use of interval training to condition for wrestling. *NSCA Strength and Conditioning Journal, 19*(5), 62-64.

13. Klinzing, J. (1986). Guidelines for conditioning in wrestling. *NSCA Strength and Conditioning Journal, 8*(2): 58-60.

14. Kovacs, M.S. (2004). A comparison of work/rest intervals in men's professional tennis. *Medicine and Science in Tennis, 9*(3), 10-11.

15. Kovacs, M.S. (2006). Applied physiology of tennis performance. *British Journal of Sports Medicine, 40*(5), 381-386.

16. Kovacs, M.S. (2007). Tennis physiology: Training the competitive athlete. *Sports Medicine, 37*(3), 1-11.

17. Kovacs, M.S., Chandler, W.B., & Chandler, T.J. (2007). *Tennis training: Enhancing on-court performance.* Vista, CA: Racquet Tech.

18. Kramer, W.J. (1984). Wrestling: Physiological aspects for conditioning. *NSCA Strength and Conditioning Journal, 40*(6), 66-67.

19. Kramer, W.J., Vescovi, J.D., & Dixon, P. (2004). The physiological basis of wrestling: Implications for conditioning programs. *NSCA Strength and Conditioning Journal, 26*(2), 10-15.

20. Manners, T.W. (2004). Sport-specific training for ice hockey. *Strength Cond J, 26*(2), 16-22.

21. McHenry, P., & Raether, J. (2004). *101 agility drills.* Monterey, CA: Coaches Choice.

22. Mero, A., & Komi, P.V. (1990). Reaction time and electromyographic activity during a sprint start. *Eur J Appl Physiol, 61,* 73-80.

23. Montgomery, D.L. (1998). Physiology of ice hockey. *Sports Medicine, 5*(2), 99-12.

24. Plisk, S.S. (2008). Speed, agility, and speed-endurance development. In T.R. Baechle & R.W. Earle, (Eds.), *Essentials of strength training and conditioning.* Champaign, IL: Human Kinetics.

25. Radcliffe, J. (2009). Trench warriors. *Training & Conditioning, 19*(3), 49-54.

26. Roetert, E.P., & Ellenbecker, T.S. (2007). *Complete conditioning for tennis* (2nd ed.). Champaign, IL: Human Kinetics.

27. Roper, R.L. (1998). Incorporating agility training and backward movement into a plyometric program. *NSCA Strength and Conditioning Journal, 20*(4), 60-63.

28. Schmidt, R.A., & Lee, T.D. (1999). *Motor control and learning: A behavioral emphasis* (3rd ed.). Champaign, IL: Human Kinetics.

29. Stucky, J. (1985). Strength and conditioning for wrestling. *NSCA Strength and Conditioning Journal, 7*(5), 40-42.

30. Twist, P. (2001). Lightning quickness. In B. Foran, (Ed.), *High-performance sports conditioning* (pp. 99-109). Champaign, IL: Human Kinetics.

31. Verstegen, M. & Marcello, B. (2001). Agility and coordination. In B. Foran (Ed.), *High-performance sports conditioning* (pp. 99-109). Champaign, IL: Human Kinetics.

32. Weber, K., Pieper, S., & Exler, T. (2007). Characteristics and significance of running speed at the Australian Open 2006 for training and injury prevention. *Medicine and Science in Tennis, 12*(1), 14-17.

33. Young, W.B., McDowell, M.H., & Scarlett, B.J. (2001). Specificity of sprint and agility training methods. *J. Strength Cond. Res., 15*(3), 315-319.

Index

Note: The italicized *f* and *t* following page numbers refer to figures and tables, respectively.

About the NSCA

The **National Strength and Conditioning Association (NSCA)** is the world's leading organization in the field of sport conditioning. Drawing on the resources and expertise of more than 30,000 professionals in strength training and conditioning, sport science, performance research, education, and sports medicine, the NSCA is the world's most trusted source of knowledge and training guidelines for coaches and athletes. The NSCA provides the crucial link between the lab and the field.

About the Editors

Jay Dawes, PhD, CSCS*D, NSCA-CPT*D, FNSCA, is an assistant professor in the department of kinesiology at Texas A& M University at Corpus Christi (TAMUCC). Before joining the TAMUCC team, Jay was the director of education for the National Strength and Conditioning Association (NSCA) and has worked as a strength and performance coach, personal trainer, educator, and postrehabilitation specialist for over 13 years. Jay is a frequent presenter, both nationally and internationally, on topics related to health, fitness, and human 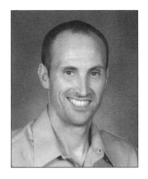 performance. He recently received his PhD from Oklahoma State University in the School of Applied Health and Educational Psychology with an emphasis in health and human performance. He is certified by the NSCA as a strength and conditioning specialist (CSCS) and as a personal trainer (NSCA-CPT), by the American College of Sports Medicine as a health fitness specialist (ACSM-HFS), and USA Weightlifting as a club coach. In addition, Jay became a fellow of the NSCA (FNSCA) in 2009.

Mark Roozen, MEd, CSCS*D, NSCA-CPT*D, FNSCA, holds a master's degree in education from Tarleton State University in Stephenville, Texas, and a bachelor's degree from Northern State University in Aberdeen, South Dakota. He is a certified strength and conditioning specialist and a certified personal trainer and has been in the strength, conditioning, and performance field for over 28 years. He has worked with teams from high school to the professional ranks as a sport coach and strength and performance coach. He was director 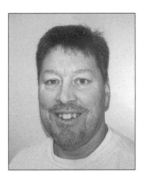 of a hospital-owned fitness and training facility and owned his own training center in Texas.

Mark is performance director for Day of Champions, which conducts sport and performance camps across the United States. He has worked with over 30,000 young men and women, including NFL greats such as Emmitt Smith, Neil Smith, Tim Dwight, and Rich Gannon. He has presented, authored, and consulted around the world for various sport and fitness groups and organizations. Mark is senior content manager for STACK Media, which promotes safe training and sport enhancement for high school and collegiate athletes. He is also codirector of The Performance Education Association (TPEA) and owner and director of Performance Edge Training Systems (PETS).

About the Contributors

Al Biancani, EdD, CSCS*D, has been working in the field of athletics and fitness for over 30 years. He received his EdD in physical education from Utah State in 1972. Al started his own strength and conditioning business in 1985 and his current business, Biancani Fitness Training, is responsible for aiding the feats of over 100 All-Americans and 150 high school all-city athletes as well as many professional athletes in baseball, basketball, football, soccer, and boxing. He is the head strength and conditioning coach for the Chinese senior women's and junior boys and girls national basketball teams.

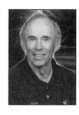

Michael Doscher, MS, CSCS*D, is currently the head strength and conditioning coach for Valdosta State University. He earned a BS degree in health fitness from Springfield College in 1992 and received his MS degree in sports administration in 1995. In 2007, he was named the Samson Division II Strength and Conditioning Coach of the Year by *American Football Monthly* while also earning the NSCA Collegiate Strength and Conditioning Professional of the Year Award in 2005.

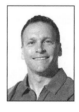

Todd Durkin, MA, CSCS, is a performance coach, personal trainer, massage therapist, and bodyworker who educates and inspires people worldwide. He earned his master's degree in exercise science from San Diego State University in 1999. Todd is the founder of Fitness Quest 10 in San Diego, named one of the top 10 gyms in the United States by *Men's Health* magazine. He trains professional, college, and high school athletes as well as regular Joes and Janes who seek optimal personal performance and overall well-being. Todd has twice been honored as Personal Trainer of the Year (IDEA and ACE), has received numerous other industry accolades, is the head of the Under Armour Performance Training Council, and is a consultant to Gatorade.

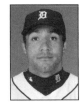

Javair Gillett, CSCS, earned his bachelor's degree in exercise science from Depauw University in 2001 and currently serves as the head strength and conditioning coach for the Detroit Tigers of Major League Baseball (MLB). Javair is also the founder of www.basesathlete.com, a website that serves as a more practical education tool for achieving healthy athletic development in youth athletes.

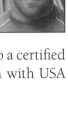

Greg Infantolino, CSCS*D, USAW, currently serves as the strength and conditioning specialist for the 3rd Special Forces Group. He previously served as the coordinator and assistant strength and conditioning coach for the NSCA Performance Center, where he was responsible for day-to-day coaching and program design for all tactical athletes. Greg is a certified strength and conditioning specialist through the NSCA. He is also a certified club coach with USA Weightlifting and a certified level I coach with USA Track and Field.

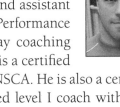

Ian Jeffreys, MSc, CSCS*D, NSCA-CPT*D, FNSCA, is a senior lecturer in strength and conditioning at the University of Glamorgan. He is the proprietor and performance director of All-Pro Performance based in Brecon, Wales. A highly experienced coach, author, and presenter, Ian has worked with athletes in a range of sports and at a range of abilities up to international level. Ian is the editor of the UKSCA journal *Professional Strength and Conditioning* and is on the editorial board for the NSCA's *Strength and Conditioning Journal* and the *Journal of Australian Strength and Conditioning*.

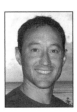

Jason Jones, MS, CSCS, has been training and assessing athletes for over 10 years. He has worked with thousands of athletes in youth, high school, and NCAA Division I to III programs in a wide range of sports. The athletes he has trained have been awarded Division I scholarships and have won the World Cup in BMX racing. Jason has also served as a consultant in establishing sport performance programs around Northern California.

Mark Kovacs, PhD, CSCS, is a performance-enhancement specialist. He combines his academic, scientific, and training backgrounds in the fields of fitness, health, wellness, nutrition, sports, and executive performance. He received a PhD in exercise physiology from the University of Alabama. Mark is a certified strength and conditioning specialist through the NSCA and a USA Track and Field level II sprint coach. In 2010 he was the recipient of the Plagenhoef Award for Sport Science Achievement.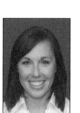

Katie Krall, LMT, CSCS*D, NSCA-CPT, USAW, earned a BS degree in kinesiology at the University of Calgary in 2003 while competing as a member of the U.S. national and World Cup speed skating teams. Currently Katie is the curriculum development coordinator for the NSCA. Upon retiring from skating in 2005, Katie became the assistant strength and conditioning coach for the NSCA Performance Center. In 2008 she completed her master's degree at the University of Colorado at Colorado Springs.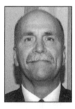

Mike Nitka, MEd, CSCS*D, FNSCA, has been the instructor of physical education at Muskego High School in Muskego, Wisconsin, since 1976. Mike earned his master's degree from the University of Wisconsin–LaCrosse and earned the NSCA fellow distinction.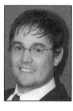

Joel Raether, MAEd, CSCS*D, is the director of sports performance for the Colorado Mammoth of the National Lacrosse League (NLL). He earned his master's of education degree in exercise science physiology from the University of Nebraska at Kearney. He is the former assistant strength and conditioning coach at the University of Denver.

Mike Sanders, MAEd, CSCS, is a human performance specialist for the Naval Special Warfare Development Group in Virginia Beach. He has worked with athletes of all levels as well as with military personnel and MMA fighters. Mike has also authored and coauthored many peer-reviewed and popular press articles related to strength and conditioning.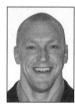

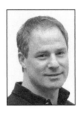

David Sandler, MS, CSCS*D, RSCC*D, FNSCA, HFI, HFD, FISSN, is the senior director of education and performance for the NSCA. David has authored six books: *Sports Power, Weight Training Fundamentals, The Resistance Band Workout Book, Plyo Power, Strength Training Everyone,* and *Fundamental Weight Training.* He has also developed dozens of exercise and developmental videos. He is a doctoral candidate at the University of Miami, where he was the assistant strength and conditioning coach and head of baseball during their 1999 National Championship season. He was an assistant professor of kinesiology and sport science for 6 years at Florida International University, where he developed and directed the strength and conditioning education curriculum before moving on to Florida Atlantic University. David has been a strength and conditioning coach and consultant for more than 20 years working with some of the world's best athletes. He was a powerlifter and three-time U.S. national bench press champion. His research focuses on strength and power development.

Jeremy Sheppard, PhD, CSCS, is the manager of athletic development and sport science at the High Performance Centre for Surfing Australia. He is also an adjunct senior lecturer for Edith Cowan University and the University of Queensland.

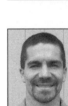

David Suprak, PhD, ATC, CSCS, has been an assistant professor of kinesiology and physical education at Western Washington University since 2008. Before this he held the following positions: assistant professor of health sciences at the University of Colorado at Colorado Springs, research and teaching assistant at the University of Oregon, and head athletic trainer and athletic training education program director at Tabor College in Hillsboro, Kansas.

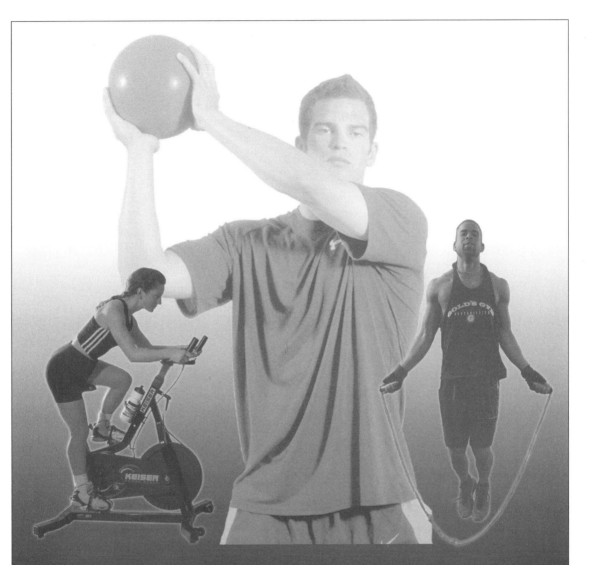
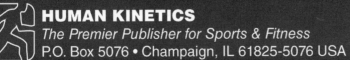
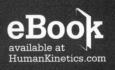